What to Tell Your Child about Sex

COMMENTARY

"Parents have an obligation to learn how to play their crucial roles as the primary sex educators of their children. This book will help them do so and may also, in the doing, help them to have better sexual lives of their own."

Mary S. Calderone, M.D.

"This little book is a classic in its field.... In a warm and human manner that is never condescending it presents authoritative sex information to assist parents with their children from infancy to adolescence. The adolescence section has been expanded and now includes the most concise and practical information on masturbation, petting, contraception, premarital intercourse and homosexuality that is currently available to parents."

Sex Information and Education Council

What to Tell Your Child about Sex

Illustrated

Prepared by the staff of

Child Study Association of America • Wel-Met Incorporated

Foreword by Mary S. Calderone, M.D.

New York • Jason Aronson • London

New Printing 1983

ISBN: 0-87668-708-7

Library of Congress Catalog Number: 84-45134

Manufactured in the United States of America.

The editorial development of this book
has been made possible through the
support of the

Helena Rubinstein Foundation, Inc.

Contents

Foreword 1

Introduction 5

I. The Early Years 11

II. Your Child from Five to Eight 27

III. Facts of Life Illustrated 35

IV. Preadolescence: Ages Nine to Twelve 43

V. The Adolescent Years: Ages Thirteen to Seventeen 55

VI. If You Need Help 83

Selected Readings for Parents, Children,
and Young People 85

Index to Questions 95

Foreword

This book is an important book. In its twenty years it has sold over a million copies, which, if you count the friends and relatives of the people who bought it, not to speak of the library borrowers, means a lot of readers.

The reason is plain: it was a ground-breaker twenty years ago—factual, objective, accurate as to the knowledge of that day, easy to read. Available at a time when good materials for parents about sex were not plentiful, it was prepared by a group of child experts connected with the highly respected and pioneering Child Study Association of America.

The original edition reflected the prevailing beliefs of the times: that telling the child the facts of human reproduction was the same thing as *educating* him about sex. Today we know that reproduction and sexuality are, even if related, two quite different areas of knowledge, feelings, and behavior. This means that we have not only learned that giving information about sex and educating the child about its uses and purposes are two quite different processes, but that *what* the child learns is less important than *how* he learns it. In other words, facts are necessary, but far more crucial to his future well-being are the attitudes that accompany that learning.

In the interval since the book was first published, research has taught us much about the sexual evolution of the human being from birth onward. We know that the child normally experiences sexual feelings very early in life, with a number spontaneously having what would appear to be orgasm in the first year. We know too that sexual feelings, curiosities, and thoughts are usual throughout childhood, and that children share these with each other if they have discovered, through painful experience, that their parents are uncomfortable, fearful, or punishing about these normal childhood experiences. Between birth and six years is when communication between parent and child about sex should be firmly established, or it may never be.

This means that the parents must first learn how to communicate with themselves and with each other about sex: How do I feel about myself as a man, a woman? About my spouse as woman or man? Do I like, fear, enjoy, dread the sex act, or am I bored with it? How does my spouse feel about these things? Can my spouse and I say vagina, penis, clitoris, masturbate, homosexual, anus, bowel movement, urinate and be comfortable about it? Can my spouse and I tell each other freely what pleases us best in lovemaking? Positive attitudes in these areas of their own private lives will enable parents to convey positive attitudes to their children about their own sexual lives, thoughts, and fantasies, which should be just as private to them.

Much marital unhappiness has its roots in negative attitudes about sexuality that were acquired in childhood, and these tend then to be passed on to the children of such marriages, thus perpetuating the sad cycle. Our nation has one of the highest divorce rates in the world about one-third higher than Sweden's. We are also a violent nation, and one whose middle-class white population has shown itself to be obsessed with sex either puritanically or exploitively. Neither extreme is healthy, and meanwhile our children beg us to give them adequate sex information and education at appropriate times in their lives, not several years too late.

Parents have an obligation to learn how to play their crucial roles as the primary sex educators of their children. This book will help them do so and may also, in the doing, help them to better sexual lives of their own.

Mary S. Calderone, M.D.
Executive Director
Sex Information and
Education Council of the U.S.

Introduction: Sex Education in a Changing World

Parents today are facing more complex challenges in rearing their children than ever before. Not least of these concerns sex education, which might more accurately be termed "human relations education." We have learned that education about sex has to be more than an extended lesson in biology. Presenting the facts of life—simply, directly, and at the appropriate time—is important. But we now know that teaching children about human sexuality involves helping them understand people and relationships, and developing in the young a sense of human values that will provide them with some guidelines for making personal choices as they approach manhood and womanhood.

Moreover, parents are expected to achieve this goal at a time when sexual mores are rapidly shifting, and they themselves are often confused and uncertain about their own values.

Confronted by the freedom of the mass media in dealing with sex—nudity on the stage and screen, the availability of pornography, the commercialization of sex to sell products on radio and TV—parents feel powerless to protect their young people from the impact of this exposure. New life-styles are being written about, talked about, experimented with, older values are being questioned. It is not surprising, then, that parents in a generation raised under vastly different conditions are shaky and uncertain.

Much of what parents teach their children is conveyed not by what they say, but by what they are and do. Children, with their acute emotional antenna, learn more about human sexuality

5

from the ways in which parents respond to each other, and to them, than from the precepts parents hand down.

How, for example, will children's perception of male and female roles be affected as their parents struggle with the changing and as yet not clearly defined concepts of femaleness and maleness? Once femaleness was equated with gentleness, nurturance, even submissiveness, and maleness with aggressiveness, competitiveness, authority, strength. Today the distinctions between the roles of male and female are blurring; young fathers may pride themselves on their nurturant functions, and young mothers on their ability to help support the family.

There is uncertainty as to how much society's expectations, and hence its educational focus, has defined the roles of boys and girls, and how much of boys' interests and girls' interests is inborn. Are little girls programmed to prefer playing with dolls and being mommies, or would they show equal interest in mechanical things if they were exposed to cars and trucks and tools as boys are? Would it influence their ultimate life goals if they were? We do not yet know the answer.

What we do know is that there are biological differences between boys and girls, that children have a deep need to know about and understand these differences from the earliest years, and that the way in which this knowledge is provided by parents, both verbal and nonverbal, can help determine the quality of "humanness" of both sexes.

This book covers the various stages of personality development in children from infancy through adolescence. It tries to weave sex into this pattern of growth rather than to treat it as a separate problem that can be dealt with in a few wholesome words of advice. The place where all emotions are first tried out is the home; here all elements of life come together through the growing-up years. No one can sift out the moment which is exclusively sexual, or separate it from other experiences.

While this book is concerned with sexual development, it would not have readers feel that their success or failure as parents can be measured by what they have done—or failed to do—in the sex education of their children. The total atmosphere created by the parents, and their whole relationship with their children and each other will be crucial in shaping the pattern of their children's development.

As a parent, therefore, you will understand that this is not a book of rules, but a guide. Being aware of the needs of children at various stages of their development, and ways of meeting these needs, is basic to their healthy sexual development. Children are likely to be flexible and responsive to honest and mutually respectful relationships.

What are my own feelings about sex? Young children have no problems about sex education. To them, sex is simply one more fascinating aspect of life to find out about. They explore and they discover.

What *do* we tell them? What are our adult standards of good and bad, helpful and harmful? Old fears and superstitions die slowly. Although we know better, and want to know more, there are ingrained adult anxieties in most of us that make us sometimes uncertain, less-than-able instructors of the young.

Parents' questions often indicate that they are baffled and embarrassed by the questions their children ask. Unthinkingly, they place adult moral values on what is—we know now—normal sexual curiosity and experimenting. And they use fear and punishment to stop it. Many parents use fables, vagueness, and untruth in telling about the great facts of conception and birth. Certainly no child ever decided on his own that he was brought by the stork or delivered in the doctor's little black bag.

Explaining the facts of life—what seems to trouble many parents most—is actually the easiest part of the job. Far more important and far more difficult is being aware of one's own attitudes and feelings.

What do I feel about myself? This is the most basic question you can ask. Love starts with appreciation of, and regard for, oneself. With growth it becomes less selfish and expands to include others. It has many variations. We can love parents, brothers, sisters, friends, sweethearts, husband or wife, children—or impersonal but nonetheless real things such as liberty, music, the sea, or nature. To love means that the lover finds worth and meaning in the loved one, thereby encouraging love in return. Happiness as a human being comes from full exercise of a wide range of emotions in both giving and receiving. But the capacity for exercising that full range of emotions is not easily attained, for incomplete growth in any stage of development is carried forward to the next stage, and lacks or failings there to the stage after that. The result, as we mature in years, is a leftover childishness in one or another area of our emotional life. Childishness means just that: underdeveloped, inexperienced feelings with which to appreciate people or situations to the fullest. The bossy husband, the spoiled, pouting wife, the man or woman who is thoughtless of the feelings of others, or careless of his responsibilities, are all obvious examples of immature behavior.

At the same time, we become so used to ourselves that we rarely take stock of our own strengths and weaknesses, to see if we really are the person we believe ourselves to be. Yet the way our children are raised is bound to be a reflection of our own feelings.

Keeping an honest eye on yourself, noting how you act and react, will make you more alert to your child's needs and better able to guide him helpfully.

What do I think about sex? Adults find it easy to give themselves credit for broad-mindedness, humor, and sensitivity—and to forget how uncomfortable they are when a child spouts four-letter words or scratches his genitals in public. These examples, of course, are not basic attitudes toward sex, but they are part of the collection of likes and dislikes that every adult has which mirror his deeper feelings.

Each person can speak only for himself about sex, and no one can tell another what he should feel. Yet to find effective ways to help children, it is important to know how you really feel about many issues. What are your feelings about menstruation? Does it embarrass or anger you to see a small child masturbate? How do you feel about intercourse outside of marriage, or before it? Do you hesitate to allow your children to play with the children of the neighbor whose male friend lives with her? Understanding that you have a point of view on a variety of such issues— and your own reasons for them—will give you a line on your feelings about the part sex plays in life.

When your child comes to you with a question, he wants the facts. But he also wants to find out what *you* think and feel. He comes to you because he trusts you; if he did not, he would have gone elsewhere. He loves you and wants to be like you; he proves this by copying you. This imitation is also applied to the invisible area of feelings. Whatever the question, words will not be answer enough unless they tell clearly what you feel.

I. The Early Years

When does sex begin? At the moment of his conception, your baby's mental and physical characteristics are established: male or female, dark or fair, large or small, placid or active. From the moment of his birth, his environment is primarily the physical, emotional, and psychological conditions provided by his parents, particularly the mother. The child's sense of security will reflect the type of care he receives: relaxed handling, tenderness, warmth will give him a sense of well-being and acceptance.

Even this early in life, his experiences build a foundation for later attitudes towards sexuality. If he senses, through the ways in which his basic bodily needs are met, that the world is good, he tends to develop feelings of trust—good feelings, pleasant feelings—which somehow seem to evolve into satisfying feelings about himself as a person.

Naturally, the change of these first bodily sensations into the complex emotions of maturity takes many years. All the steps are linked, however, and none is more important than those he takes in his first year, even before he has spoken his first word.

What does baby learn first? Once he has begun to breathe, baby's efforts and feelings are keyed to the satisfaction of his appetite. With his first strong reflex action—sucking—he learns to feed himself at breast or bottle. Above all, this eases his hunger pangs and keeps him alive. But before long it is also a pleasure. He gurgles and sighs at the delightful feeling of being full after the discomfort of being empty. Often he wants to go on sucking even though it is plain he couldn't hold another drop. Between feedings he sucks his fingers or a toy.

Through sucking, too, he makes his first contact with another person. This is an important relationship. The way he feels about it will help to shape his later attitudes toward people generally. If, for instance, he is soothingly held while feeding he will feel the warmth of human affection and will be encouraged, as he grows, to express warmth to others. By contrast, the baby who is not sufficiently touched, held, and caressed, or who is left alone in his crib most of the time, may indeed suffer serious physical and emotional consequences as a result of such deprivation.

Can an unhappy experience at this age do permanent damage? Probably no single everyday experience—happy or unhappy—has a permanent effect. Children do not grow up loving mankind because their bottles are on time or hating it because they are late. But it *is* true that patterns of feeling start to form very early around the simple events of a baby's life. This does not mean that baby must—or can—be protected from upsets. What matters is that he is loved and cared for. Babies do differ in their capacity to tolerate frustrations or traumatic experiences. Nevertheless, all babies need the bodily contact and warmth that comes from being fondled and talked to.

Babies do sense tension or anger in those caring for them, but occasional moods will not seriously affect them. A continuing atmosphere of anxiety or tension may, however, set up a corresponding feeling in the baby.

Should baby be stopped from putting everything in his mouth? Parents are naturally concerned when baby begins to put everything in his mouth. As months go by, the mouth becomes baby's chief means of testing new elements in his world. Whatever comes to hand is thrust into the mouth to explore its characteristics and to see if it will stir up the pleasure sensations he has learned are there. Since he doesn't know enough to choose, many of the items he puts in his mouth may be odd or even dangerous, and certainly not to your liking. At the same time, he is not likely to agree that he is better off for having an object taken away from him. As far as he is concerned, he has simply been prevented from enjoying himself.

Sucking is a natural activity for infants and need not be a problem if the child is given opportunities and freedom to suck on objects that are safe.

When does sucking stop? Usually when the youngster becomes interested in trying out his surroundings and using his hands in other ways. This is not so much a matter of age as of personality growth. As a child advances to new activities, such as playing with other children or with toys that he enjoys manipulating (blocks, cars, dolls, trucks), he begins to drop more babyish habits. Of course, the process is rarely clean-cut. Few children suddenly give up sucking forever. For most, there will be times of tiredness or unhappiness, well into the preschool years or even later, when it seems easier to be a baby again and to return to the comfort of sucking.

Of all baby habits, thumb sucking seems to bother parents most. It doesn't look very bright, and it raises the fear that baby's teeth and jaws will be deformed. Since no parent wants that, firm treatment is often used to stop it.

Actually, harsh measures just don't work, and they may be harmful and reinforce the problem. While experts disagree on the dangers of thumb sucking, most studies seem to show that no harm will be done if the youngster has stopped sucking before he begins to get his second teeth.

It is generally recognized that some children are born with greater needs for sucking than others, and whether breast or bottle fed will continue to suck thumbs—or other fingers or pacifiers—oftener and longer than children with less urgent sucking needs. (Some fetuses, for example, have been photographed in the uterus with thumbs in mouth.) If a child continues to suck fingers actively into the school years, teasing by other children about being a baby often provides the motivation for him to give it up. Parents can also try to motivate him to stop by encouraging his own efforts to stop through praise and recognition, but should never do so by shaming or humiliating.

Is masturbation dangerous? No, not in the sense that generations of parents have worried about. It definitely does not lead to ailments or injuries of any kind and is generally regarded as a normal part of sexual development.

Masturbation begins in young children as the result of natural interest in touching and finding out about their bodies. They soon discover that there is a pleasant, enjoyable feeling to be had from touching or rubbing the genitals, and so they do it, to the great distress of some parents.

Masturbation does not cause insanity, skin blemishes, blindness, poor sexual adjustment in adult life, or any of the other troubles parents are frightened about. What can happen, however, is that a child may develop unhealthy feelings of anxiety and guilt, especially if he has been scolded or punished for masturbating. This is a real threat to mental health; masturbation in itself is not. If your child has other interests, the masturbating can be ignored.

Children need to know quite early that masturbation is something that is not generally accepted as public behavior. Every person growing up needs to know what is acceptable as private as distinguished from public behavior. And behavior that is "private" doesn't mean it is "bad."

And don't try to talk it out, even sympathetically. Usually, a child doesn't want to talk with parents about masturbation—and he shouldn't be forced to. If he feels that you enjoy him and like to do things with him, very likely he will sense a kind of support and understanding that is more valuable than verbal reassurance.

Very early the child begins to explore his body. Even as he discovered his fingers and toes, so he will discover his genitals and want to touch them. This is quite normal, completely innocent, and to be expected. At the same time, he is likely to become interested in urination and bowel movements. He will want to see the size of his stools, may want to handle them, and far from being disturbed, may even enjoy soiled clothing. He will also be curious about the toilet habits of other children.

For adults with feelings of privacy about bathroom functions, the primitive interests of the child may be trying. Yet, this, too, is a chance to guide him toward a comfortable, healthy pattern of perceiving himself. The attitude toward physical functions that you pass on to him will be one basis for his feeling good about himself and the way his body works.

What about toilet training? Many of your child's feelings about himself will be formed as you begin the process of toilet training. As with most learning, your success will depend upon your ability to see what is involved from the child's point of view. For the child it is a difficult physical process to bring the untrained muscles of bowel and bladder under control, and it cannot be mastered until his muscles and his nervous system are mature enough. Since the child may not know or care that he's being messy, control may mean giving up a familiar pleasure in order to gain your approval.

A child's impulse to please the people he loves is strong. Yet his abilities may not equal his intentions. Bear with him. Make your training gentle and gradual. Help him to understand what you want him to do and avoid showing displeasure when he fails. He needs your patience and warm approval to feel that the struggle is worthwhile.

It is important during this training that he should not get the feeling from you that any part of him is bad or dirty. Long before he understands words he will be sensitive to looks, gestures, and tones of voice. For his parents to suggest that some parts of him or his functions are not "nice" may raise doubt, confusion, and anxiety in him. This is especially important because he may associate his toilet functions with his sex organs.

When is he ready to start? Children are ready to begin learning control of their bowel functions before they can start learning bladder control. Control of elimination involves the whole nervous system as well as a set of muscles—called sphincters. In addition, the child must be mature enough to understand what is expected of him. His muscles must be developed to the point where they can be consciously controlled at the proper time. As his eliminations become more regular—which usually happens between fifteen months and two years—he is ready to be trained, and will be far better able to cooperate and far more willing. Readiness to begin using a potty for urinating may be indicated when the child can hold his urine for several hours during the day. However it may be some time before he is completely dry during the day, and even longer before nighttime dryness can be achieved. If he can see that his own efforts are helping in his training, he will take greater pride in his accomplishment and will be less likely to slip back into soiling or wetting later on. A relaxed, loving approach will make the child feel that his parents want to help him in his efforts.

Must we use "scientific" words? Parents often find it hard to give names to the various parts and functions of the body, being content to use the words of their own childhood. There is no reason not to be content although eventually a child will need to know the proper terms—urine, bowel movements, vagina, penis, and so on—it will certainly do no harm to let him know them early. As a matter of fact, they are not easy words to pronounce, and he will need some time to get used to them.

Should a child see his parents nude? To begin with, at one time or another he probably will. Nudity embarrasses many adults and may spur them to say something abrupt, which leaves the child feeling he shouldn't have asked about it. The child is blamed for having natural curiosity, and he gets a sense of guilt. One good way for children to learn about nudity is to allow them to see other children.

Some grown-ups today make a point of going nude in front of their children, believing that it's best to be natural and that it helps give the young ones a wholesome, matter-of-fact feeling toward the body. Actually, this isn't always so. Seeing the nude bodies of grown-ups may arouse a child's interest in touching, exploring, or fondling. This may be sexually stimulating and start feelings and desires in him that can't be satisfied. Some children show this clearly. With others you can't be sure. Parents need to be alert to how their own children are reacting and to do what seems most comfortable for them.

Should I let my child into the bathroom with me? Surely you are entitled to this privacy if you wish it, and this is something children learn quite easily. However, the toilet habits of an adult can help to give a small child an idea of bodily functions and of the way they are performed. Small boys may be shown by fathers how to urinate. Once a child's own toilet habits are established, however, there is certainly no need to have him in the bathroom as an observer. If at times he beats on the door and insists on being let in, it usually has something to do with a feeling of being shut out. If the child seems worried by your absence, you can tell him, "Wait for me—I'll be with you in a minute," before you leave him.

Does it help to use examples of sex in nature? It is part of the life experience for children to observe the habits of animals, including their mating. If these observations lead them to ask questions, adults must be prepared to answer them. However, when a child asks about the structure of his body, or about how babies are born, it's human experience he's interested in. To be

answered with talk about bees and flowers is confusing and eva-
sive.

With older children, who have an accurate fund of knowledge
to work from, the habits of other living things will be of interest
and can broaden their knowledge of life processes.

Does the father have a place in sex education? It is important for
the growing child to have a clear view of each sex as a guide to
his own behavior as a male or female. For both boys and girls,
fathers provide a model of maleness that they need.

There is also the fact that sometime in these early years children often feel attracted to the parent of the opposite sex, and
may feel as a result a sense of disloyalty toward the parent of the
same sex. A boy at times will express a desire to "marry mommy,"
and at other times will swing to daddy's side to be like him and
to assure himself of his father's love.

Little girls usually reverse the situation, wanting to "marry
daddy" and ignoring mommy, and then wanting, as a girl, to be
like her.

At this age children will begin to identify themselves primarily
with the parent of their own sex. A boy will imitate his father
and a girl will want to be like her mother. For this reason, it is
important for both parents to give the youngster something to
pattern themselves after. Parents need to be alert to the nature
of the emotional pull-and-tug going on and to help the child deal
with the conflict. Go easy on romping and roughhouse that involve too much intimate physical contact, and do not encourage
the child to become a substitute for his or her parent of the same
sex. More than this, both parents should try to show that they are
united in their unwavering affection for the child.

What if there is no father in the home? Naturally, mothers who
are rearing children alone have an additional task. Where parents
are separated or divorced, it is helpful for children to maintain

their relationship with their father, so long as he is available to them. If he has no contact with them, the mother should be careful not to downgrade him before the children. It is hard for a little boy to identify with the male role if his mother is constantly expressing dislike for men, or for a little girl to develop respect for males under such circumstances. If the father does have some contact with the children, it is thought best for the children to know him, whether he is a good model or not, as they will eventually have to make their own decision as to whether they will choose him as a male model or choose another male as a model.

It is particularly important for the lone mother not to use the little boy as a substitute for the missing mate—to tell him that he is the "man of the house" and cuddle and take him into her bed. This can create considerable anxiety and guilt.

Most mothers alone do have some relatives or friends nearby, and can encourage male cousins, uncles, friends to show an interest in, and spend time with, her children. Children often develop deep bonds with men who are not their natural fathers, and adopt them as their role models.

How can I talk about sex comfortably? There *is* a special quality of intimacy, of significance, about sex, and this makes it difficult for many people to deal with it comfortably. Even small children recognize this and sense our discomfort. It is important to recognize one's own feelings honestly and to be as candid with children as possible. If you find it impossible to do this, it might be desirable to ask for help from some person close to the family. Here are some guidelines:

1. Be patient. It is hard to grow up. Children grope and fumble and make many trial starts before they make forward progress. Don't rush them. Be prepared to have the same questions come up over and over again, without answering, "But I told you."

2. Be a good listener. It is important to know *what* your child really wants to know; try to respond to *his* question. The three or four year old who wants to know where he comes from is not necessarily curious about sexual intercourse or childbirth. More than likely he is concerned with finding out about his own origins and with strengthening his feeling of belonging. Don't overwhelm him with all you know. Encourage him to say what he believes is the answer to his question. Listening, after all, is part of mutual give-and-take. Keep a clear channel open between you and your questioner so that you can understand each other.

3. Keep your terms simple. Gear your answers to the child's level of experience and understanding.

4. Be honest and be consistent. This is especially important when husband and wife, or other family members or care-takers, are likely to be asked questions by the youngsters and may have varied points of view. Knowing generally the age at which one type of question or another may be raised, you might come to an understanding of how you would handle the questions. It doesn't hurt a child to know that there is more than one way of looking at things; nevertheless he'll be less confused if he gets consistent answers to basic questions.

It is not necessary to pretend that you know all the answers. Sooner or later the child will discover that you don't; it will help if you know and accept this too. Your own sensitivity to your child's needs will be your best guide in answering his questions. By observing him you will get some clues as to what his queries mean. To the degree that you are frank and open with him you will be giving him more opportunity to communicate with you.

What are some of the questions preschool children ask? As we have already said, sex education starts in intangible ways almost at birth. By the age of three or four, when he is talking and active enough to take an interest in his own body and those of the people around him, he generally begins to ask specific questions.

This development comes as part of his general interest in the family group and his growing awareness of similarities and differences among them. He will note that his mother looks different from his father in several respects, that little girls are equipped differently than little boys, that people about him have different skin and hair color. It is perfectly natural that he should wonder about these obvious differences.

Be prepared to handle questions whenever they come up, and try not to postpone them. Small children have almost no time sense and "later" is the same as no answer at all. He will have forgotten what he wanted to know by the time you are ready to discuss it, and may get the sense that the question is taboo.

At some point boys and girls will notice that their genitals are different, and they will ask about it. The answer that usually suffices is that boys (and grown-up men) have a penis and girls (and grown-up women) have a vagina. In families where there are numerous boys and only one girl, or numerous girls and only one boy, the lone child tends to feel *very* different. But children as a rule have little difficulty in accepting this difference, provided they know their parents accept and love them as a boy or as a girl.

Small boys may be concerned about the size of their father's (or older brothers or cousins) sex organs compared with their own. However, pointing out that fathers are bigger all over, and that the child's genitals will grow as he grows usually makes sense to them.

Preschool children will also notice their navels and wonder what they are for. This can often provide parents with an opportunity to explain that a baby grows inside the mother's body, in a uterus, and that while the baby is there a cord from her body to his gives him nourishment until he is ready to be born. The navel is where that cord was attached to him.

Having learned about babies growing inside the mother's body, children may become concerned about how babies survive without air. "How does the baby breathe inside the mother?" may be an anxious or curious question. All that is needed are a few reassuring remarks that babies get air through the same cord that provides their food, until they get outside the mother's body.

Some youngsters may also ask, in the same vein, "How does the baby go to the bathroom inside the mother?" The answer is the same—through the cord that attaches baby and mother.

Children often become confused when parents are vague about where the uterus is or refer to the baby as growing "in the mother's stomach." They may then confuse the idea of conception with the digestive process, and have been known to develop eating difficulties due to subtle fears of having a baby grow in their stomachs. Similarly, talking about reproduction in terms of a "seed growing inside mommy" may also give a child the mistaken notion that birth is part of a digestive process. It's best to be accurate here, and use the proper terms, such as "uterus" instead of "stomach."

Sooner or later, children want to know how a baby gets out of his mother's body: "Where does the baby come out?" Usually this question comes when the child is ready for this information, and your answer need not be volunteered earlier or postponed until later. Tell your child that the baby comes out of a special opening in the mother's body, called a vagina, or birth canal, between her thighs. This serves as a passageway into the world from the place where the baby has been growing.

Children may not always understand that in a woman there are three different openings. If they wonder about it, you might add that just in front of the vagina is an opening, the urethra, for urination.

Occasionally a child will ask to see the "place where I came out." This is natural curiosity, but most parents will realize that it is unwise to satisfy this wish. You can simply say you'd rather not, but you will tell him whatever he wants to know. This can also be an opportunity to use the simple biological diagrams in this book, or in other books for children, which show the human reproductive process (see p. 36).

Children frequently ask, "Does it hurt to have a baby?" They can be told that it may hurt some while the baby is being born; some mothers learn special exercises that help lessen any pain and some are given special pain relievers. This may be a good opportunity to explain the birth process in a simple way. Explain that when the baby is ready to be born, the uterus helps the process with a pushing motion. The mother feels these muscles working and knows that the baby is getting ready to come out. She may go to the hospital to have her baby, so that a doctor can help, but this doesn't mean she is sick but that she needs to be in a place where she can get the right care, and, if she needs it, to make the birth less painful.

"Why can't men have babies?" They weren't meant to. Men's bodies have no special place (uterus) where a baby can grow and no passageway (birth canal) to let a baby come into the world. Their part is to help start the baby by planting the sperm in the mother's body, and to take care of the mother and baby later.

"Why do women have breasts?" Breasts make the milk that feeds little babies. Some mothers feed their babies that way before they are ready for a bottle or cup. Little girls get breasts as they grow up; little boys don't.

What if a child never asks questions about sex? It is unusual for a child to reach the age of four without having some questions about the differences between the sexes or about the human reproductive process. Even an only child is likely to have seen a pregnant relative or neighbor, and most children have watched a baby of the opposite sex being diapered. If a child never asks questions about these things, it may mean that he has gotten the feeling that such questions are off limits in his home. Perhaps he has often asked questions, but indirectly, and the parent has not understood it for what it was, or tuned it out because he or she wasn't quite ready to answer it.

When a child does not seem to ask questions spontaneously, parents may have to think about ways to introduce the subject—perhaps arranging to watch a new baby being bathed or changed, or commenting on a neighbor's expanding figure with a casual "she's going to have a baby."

Are books helpful in talking to young children? There are a number of good books for children of various ages which can be read to them by parents, but only to supplement what the parent has already said in her own words. Some of the pictures and diagrams of the human body can help clarify what the parent has been saying. (See p. 36 for suggestions.)

II. Your Child From Five to Eight

In this period, children's views of the world are greatly widened. They leave home for school, and although family ties are still very strong, they make new contacts with other people who become important to them. Teachers, schoolmates, parents of friends will offer information and points of view that help shape children's outlook on life. They begin to read books, magazines, comic books. They become more aware of the implications of what they see on TV.

Their bodies grow and strengthen; they begin to use their muscles better, not only in games and play, but gradually in writing, drawing pictures, or playing musical instruments. Through being in groups, they learn to give and take, and to share somewhat more graciously. They gain a clearer idea of the results of their own behavior and how this affects their relations with other people. They work hard to understand the facts of their ever-widening world—what is so and why it is so. Their sense of time and space improves; they ask questions about the past and the future as well as the present. They are learning more about themselves— what they like, what they dislike—and are finding out how to become more of an individual. They begin to make some choices about what they will do, with whom, and when. Naturally, they still need firm support and direction from parents, but letting them make some decisions for themselves, in some matters, gives them some practice for making more difficult choices in the future.

Perhaps because the growth hormones have become more active, and the sex hormones less so, or because they are more involved in a variety of interests and activities, children at this age seem less obviously interested in sexual matters. Nevertheless, some may go in for childish sex play, such as looking at or touching other children's genitals or telling "dirty" jokes. They may disappear into the bathroom with their friends, where they may explore each others genitals or even play at stimulating each other. Sometimes these indoor sports take the form of playing "hospital" or "doctor," which gives them a somewhat more socially acceptable way to do the same things. Occasionally children overdo these activities, and may even be troubled by them, without knowing quite how to get out of the situation. Here is where the parent needs to step in and take charge without making a fuss or becoming angry and punitive. A clearly meant "no" to undressing games or group trips to the bathroom, or too long, too quiet play behind closed doors may actually serve to relieve children from dealing with a situation that has gotten out of hand. They may welcome a suggestion of some other activity.

At this age, too, children may begin to exchange the kinds of sex "misinformation" that confuses and troubles them so much. If they do ask any questions about human reproduction and sexual relations—and they may seem to be the same questions they asked you earlier—now is the time to give them straight factual answers and possibly also a book geared to their age and reading level, with encouragement to ask you about anything they don't understand. This does not mean that they need or want a lot of detail about lovemaking, or complex adult emotional states. Stay within the framework of the questions they are asking and don't offer information that hasn't been asked for.

What are some of the questions children from five to eight ask? A natural follow-up to the first questions children ask about where they came from is: "How does a baby get inside the mother?" Five and six year olds may be content to be told that the father must start the baby growing inside the mother. If your child wants to know more, you can explain that a fluid called semen, containing many tiny sperm cells, comes from the father's body. One cell joins an egg cell in the mother's body. The joining of these two cells starts the growth of the baby.

"How do the mother and father cells get together?" The semen containing the male sperm cells comes out through the father's penis. When the man puts his penis into the woman's vagina, this is called sexual intercourse, or mating. This explanation may not be fully absorbed by the child at this point. It may even strike him as odd, since he knows that his father urinates through his penis. This may lead to the natural query, "Is semen the same as urine?" The answer, of course, is no. Semen is a special fluid whose only purpose is to carry the male sperm cells from the testicles, where they are formed, to the outside of the body. Urine, which is a body waste, uses the same passageway through the penis, but it comes from a storage sac called the bladder and never comes out at the same time as semen.

Some children by this age may be aware that something special goes on in the parental bedroom. They may very well ask, "When do a mother and father mate?" but not be all that interested in any details. Perhaps the simplest reply is, "When they are alone."

By this time, children are alert to the signs of pregnancy in the family or neighborhood, and may well ask, "Why does the mother get so big?" Explain that the baby grows inside the mother until he is big enough to come into the world. The uterus in which he grows is made of muscle and can stretch a great deal to make room for him. Fluid also forms inside the uterus to float the baby and protect him from bumps and jolts.

A child may also ask again, "How does the baby get out?" He can be told that there is a passageway (vagina, birth canal) in the mother's body that can expand to permit the baby to come out. After the baby is born, the mother becomes her usual size again. "How big is a baby when he's born?" he may inquire. Usually about six or seven pounds, sometimes more, sometimes less. You may add that if a baby arrives much earlier than he should and is very small, he may need special care.

Should fathers as well as mothers be involved in sex education?
Of course fathers are involved in the sex education of their children. They are involved by the ways in which they relate to all the family members, demonstrated by their kindness, warmth, and affection, their concern for their mate and children, or the lack of these. If they are involved in activities with their children, they are more readily available for the spontaneous kinds of questions that grow naturally out of doing things together. Under these conditions children may find it just as easy to communicate with their fathers as their mothers, in some cases easier. Many a girl has been told about menstruation by a sympathetic father when she found it hard to talk to her mother, and boys often feel more comfortable talking about the male role in sex with their fathers.

Where the father is not in the home, a male relative or family friend sometimes becomes the person to whom the child can turn.

Should children share a bed or bedroom? Children who regularly share a bed are necessarily thrown into close physical contact and it is not unusual for this to lead to some sex play, even between brothers, sisters, or brother and sister. Where it is possible, it is a good idea to avoid the stimulation that close physical proximity inevitably sets up. If it can be managed, male and female siblings should not sleep in the same room. If such separation is not possible, some other arrangements might be made to provide privacy.

Sharing a bedroom with parents is not desirable. Children aren't always asleep when they seem to be and may be disturbed by the sounds of parental sexual activity. A baby's crib can be rolled into another room when parents retire. If there is only one bedroom, many couples prefer to sleep on a sofa bed and let the children have the bedroom.

Should children be told about child molesters? Parents are understandably alarmed by newspaper reports or neighborhood incidents of sexual violence to children, yet hesitate to warn children to beware of strangers lest children become overly fearful. The realities of life, however, make it necessary for parents to alert children who are old enough to walk the city streets or suburban roads by themselves about possible offbeat encounters. They can be told, with as little fuss as possible, that they must always refuse offers to accompany strangers, whether in cars or on foot. Most children by age seven or eight have seen the frightening results of such encounters on television programs or heard about rape and kidnapping on the news broadcasts. Suggestions that they travel in groups rather than alone and keep to the more populated streets and parks are a few precautions. They can also be told to avoid reacting to exhibitionists, whose need is to shock, and to seek protection in the nearest well-populated neighborhood store or the company of known neighborhood adults. Later, they should be warned to stay away from public washrooms, movies, or park areas where disturbed loners loiter.

If, despite precautions, a child should experience a sexual advance, whether by a stranger or an adult known to the family (perhaps even a relative), it is important for the parent to remain as calm as possible. Children need comfort and reassurance under such circumstances. Hysterical reactions by parents can be more upsetting than the experience itself. Children can be questioned later about what happened, and care should be taken to do this sensitively. Except for tragic accidents, the prevention of sexual molestation depends to a great extent on adequately preparing a child to be aware of dangers, to behave discriminately, and to avoid taking unnecessary chances.

What is the parent's role during the five-to-eight period? This is a time when parents need to recognize the fact that their child's life is beginning to include other people and other influences besides those in the home. Nevertheless, home is still the most important factor in their lives, and parents are still their major source of values.

It is a time when parents can encourage the child's widening interests by making new activities available to him, encouraging his own sense of competence and mastery of new skills, and wherever possible participating in activities with him. Paying attention to his expressions of thought and ideas will enable him to stay in communication with you.

III. Facts of Life Illustrated

THE MALE

His sex organs produce and deliver the active sperm cells which fertilize the female ovum to start new life.

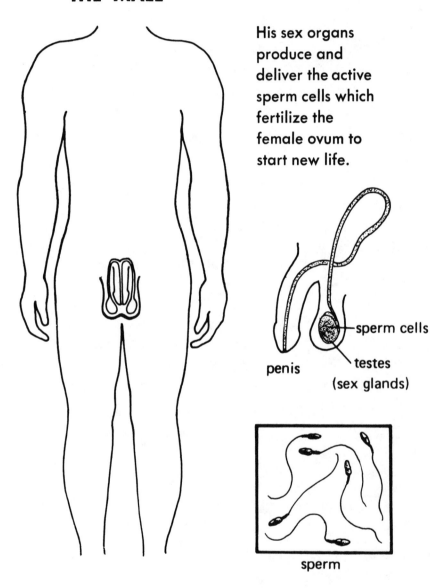

sperm cells

penis

testes (sex glands)

sperm

THE FEMALE

Her delicately
balanced sexual
system renews
itself each month
in preparation
for the role
of motherhood.

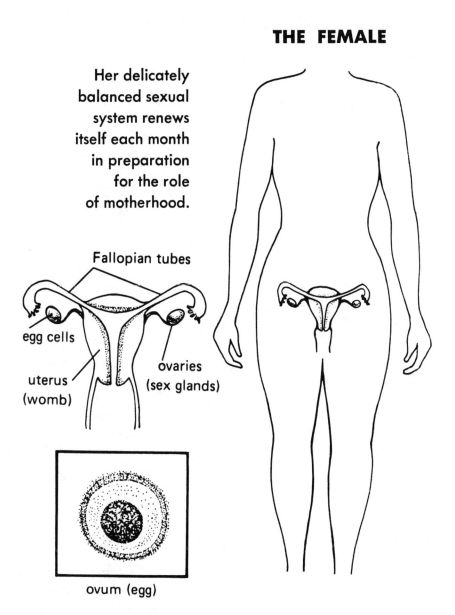

Fallopian tubes

egg cells

uterus
(womb)

ovaries
(sex glands)

ovum (egg)

THE BEGINNING OF LIFE

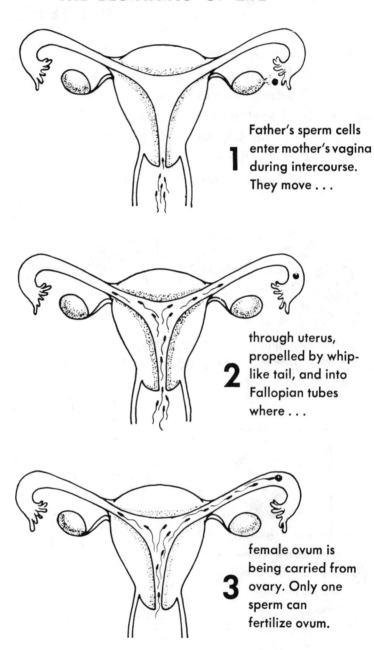

1 Father's sperm cells enter mother's vagina during intercourse. They move . . .

2 through uterus, propelled by whip-like tail, and into Fallopian tubes where . . .

3 female ovum is being carried from ovary. Only one sperm can fertilize ovum.

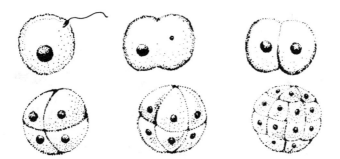

4 Growth begins. Fertile cell subdivides many times. Each one has chromosomes which determine physical characteristics.

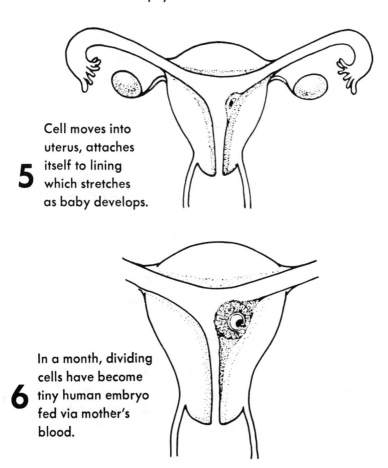

5 Cell moves into uterus, attaches itself to lining which stretches as baby develops.

6 In a month, dividing cells have become tiny human embryo fed via mother's blood.

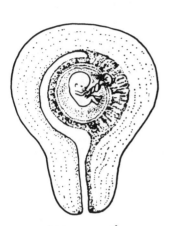

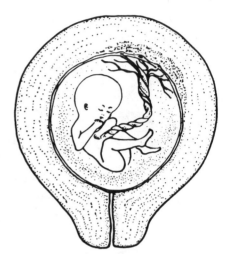

7 At two months, embryo is only an inch long but form is human. He floats . . .

8 in "bag of waters," is nourished, by fourth month has become four-ounce fetus.

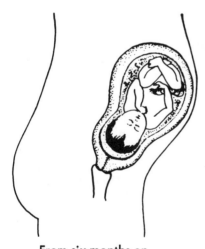

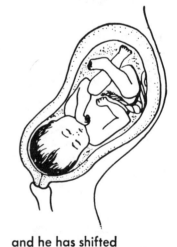

9 From six months on, baby's presence is very noticeable. Mother can feel movement . . .

10 and he has shifted into head-down position in which he likely will be born.

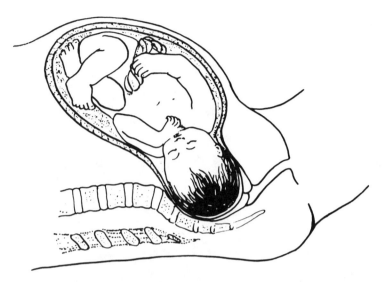

11 Birth begins sometime in ninth month. Muscles of uterus contract to help push baby out, waters ease . . .

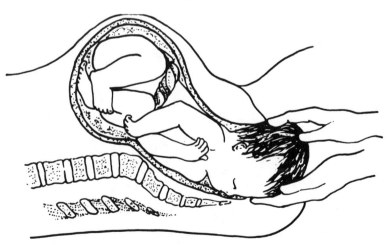

12 passage into world. With assist from doctor, baby becomes air-breathing member of human race.

IV. Preadolescence: Ages Nine to Twelve

This is a period when the first real, if tentative, drive to become an independent person begins. It is a trial run, so to speak, of the later, more specific drive for independence of the adolescent.

One's own peer group, or age-mates, become a source of finding one's identity in new ways, unlike those learned in the home. Clubs, sports, extracurricular school acitivities, and being with the crowd, usually of the same sex, becomes more important than being with one's family.

This is a time that tries the patience and understanding of even the best parents. For in preadolescence—roughly the period from nine to twelve years of age—many children begin to flaunt the rules and regulations which their parents have taught them. They are often rude, sloppy, noisy, and disobedient. They tease their siblings, are rarely on time, don't like to bathe, pay attention, or sit still. They bicker among themselves and challenge adult ideas.

It is important during these years for boys to develop solid relationships with other boys, and for girls to form close relationships with other girls. These friendships, with their concomitant sharing of interests and activities are as necessary to social development as the later close relationships with members of the opposite sex.

With earlier physical maturation and the many stimuli from the mass media, many boys and girls—particularly girls, who mature even more rapidly than boys—do feel pushed into early dating and even "going steady," which for many really means having someone they can count on to take them to the movies and be seen with. It's certainly all right for parents to encourage young people to share mutual interests and activities, such as bicycling, playing tennis, going bowling, listening to records, and dancing, especially if these can be arranged as group activities. Few youngsters of this age are really ready for the emotional wear and tear of premature dating or the too-early sexual involvement that close attachment may foster.

Mostly, though, in the early years of preadolescence, both boys and girls are involved in the special subculture of their peers of the same sex, with whom they develop the games, rituals, loyalties that purposely shut out adults. The child begins to test out his own skills, competence, and values and start to look at himself more realistically as an individual outside of the family. Much of his time and effort outside of school is devoted to acquiring the major and minor motor skills that his developing body makes possible, and boys and girls alike are involved in physical sports, music lessons, dancing lessons, and club activities.

Parents often feel caught in a bind at this juncture in their children's lives, since they quite rightly feel that sex is a highly sensitive subject to discuss with young people of this age. At the same time, they are increasingly aware that through the mass media children are becoming much more familiar with sexual matters and that there are many pressures toward precocity in this area. Also, the preadolescent, with his greater wariness about expressing his feelings to his parents and his increased awareness of adult taboos, is less likely than the younger child to ask specific questions. Yet the realistic parent knows quite well that he is picking up information, misinformation (and more of the latter than the former), and attitudes from his friends. The recognition that the child needs to be prepared for the overt physical changes that are soon to occur and that it is easier to provide necessary information while it is primarily of informational interest and before the young person is embroiled in the emotional stresses of adolescence, often enables parents to deal with it directly. Sometimes, though, it is easier for the child to ask questions of an adult who is not his parent—a health education teacher in the school, a club leader, or camp counselor—and some parents prefer to have this happen, particularly if they know and trust this person. Parents who feel it important to inculcate a sense of their own values toward sexual matters may take the initiative in raising the subject if their children don't.

What about masturbation? Masturbation, the manipulation of the genitals to achieve erotic arousal, is believed to be practiced by almost all males and a great many females. Many practice it from infancy and early childhood, but it reaches a peak during adolescence.

While it is now widely recognized that it can cause no physical harm, it may create anxiety among those young people whose religious or family backgrounds have led them to feel it is wrong or dangerous. The erotic fantasies accompanying masturbation may also disturb such young people, unless they can be assured that these, too, are a normal part of this aspect of sexual development.

Eventually most young people have less need to masturbate as they find outlets for their sexual urges in sexual activity with others. Yet many married men and women, or adults whose sexual activities have been curtailed by lack of a sexual partner, may find a normal release of sexual tensions in masturbation even in their later years. For some adults masturbation is a part of their sexual expression throughout their entire life.

What do preadolescents know about sexual development? Since girls mature physically earlier than boys, by the age of nine they should be prepared for what those changes will be. Most girls and some boys will already know something about menstruation, even if their parents have not discussed it with them, as they will have seen and heard advertisements for the sanitary pads, tampons, and menstrual pain-relievers and will have been curious about them. Very often boys will have speculated about the uses of these devices with their pals, as will girls, but very few of them will have clear or accurate information.

What is menstruation? The word menstruation means "monthly flow," and it describes one part of the complex cycle by which the female body prepares itself every twenty-eight days or so for the conception and birth of a child.

Each month an egg cell, or ovum, matures in one of the woman's two ovaries, the oval-shaped organs located at either side of her uterus, or womb, in the lower abdomen. When one of the egg cells leaves the ovary, it finds its way to the fallopian tubes, one of which serves each ovary and leads to the uterus. This process is called ovulation. When the egg is fertilized by a male sperm cell in sexual intercourse, it travels down the tube and attaches itself to the wall of the uterus. Here it begins the complicated process of development into a baby. In preparation for the possibility that fertilization might occur, the lining of the uterus has thickened with an extra supply of nourishing blood.

If fertilization does not take place, however, the uterus has no need for the lining (or endometrium) and it is cast off. This is the flow of blood and tissue from the vagina that happens during menstruation.

Each month the same cycle occurs. When it starts and how long it lasts may vary widely. In young girls the monthly periods may be irregular for some time. Eventually, however, they usually take place every twenty-eight days, and last from three to six days.

Even before the first flow, which may begin as early as nine or ten years of age, most girls are interested in the practical details of what happens and how. A woman's own attitudes toward menstruation will naturally influence the way in which she presents these facts. If she has felt it to be a "curse"—as women often referred to the monthly flow in the past—or a "sick time," she will tend to pass on these views to her children, much as the old misconceptions and taboos that surrounded it were passed on to her. Today, young women and girls are more likely to speak of it as their "monthly period" and to accept it simply as a basic aspect of being a woman. Many girls today look forward eagerly to the beginning of the menstrual cycle as their initiation into the joys and mysteries of womanhood.

Before menstruation starts, a girl should be prepared to deal with it. She should be told how to wear sanitary pads or tampons that can be inserted into the vagina without disturbing the hymen, how to insure cleanliness, how much exercise to take, and what to do for the discomfort, if any, that she may have. Today most girls continue their usual activities during their monthly periods, since there is no medical reason why they cannot, although some doctors discourage swimming in cold water.

Does ovulation or menstruation hurt? Usually menstruation does not cause pain. Some girls have menstrual cramps, which can be relieved by a mild pain killer and rest. If the cramps are severe, and interfere with a girl's normal activities, she should be checked by a physician, preferably a gynecologist, to determine whether this is due to some condition that can be corrected.

While a positive attitude toward menstruation and acceptance of her femaleness help offset any physical discomforts, there can be a tendency to feel "blue" when a period is about to start. This condition is referred to as "menstrual tension" and is related to a lowered level of hormonal secretions, leading to a let-down feeling.

Teaching boys to know why girls act touchy and out-of-sorts on certain days, and the physiological reasons for this may help them be more understanding. Girls should be given the facts about the functioning of the male sexual system.

For both sexes, answering their questions about menstruation can open the way for an honest and thorough discussion of all their questions about the human reproductive process. Both parents and young people can be aided in this discussion by referring to some of the many books available on this subject for both adults and young people. (See p. 84 for suggestions.)

Why do boys have wet dreams? Preadolescent boys do not have to be prepared for a sexual change as dramatic as menstruation. But they should be told of the changes that will affect them sometime after age twelve. They should know that wet dreams are emissions of semen that occur involuntarily from time to time, usually during the night. These nocturnal emissions are normal —as are the sexual dreams and fantasies that accompany them— and most boys have them.

Discussion of nocturnal emissions may spark some questions about sexual intercourse. You can explain that during sexual intercourse, or the physical act of mating, the man's penis increases in length, becomes stiff, and stands up at an angle from the body. This is an erection. It enables the male to insert the penis into the female vagina, where the sperm cells, mixed with fluid, are ejaculated.

How do the male organs of sex and reproduction work? Male sperm cells—one of which has to meet and unite with a woman's egg cell for reproduction to take place—are produced in the testicles, or testes. These are two oval glands, each about one and one-half inches long, enclosed in a kind of sac of loose skin, called the scrotum, which hangs below the body.

The testes, like all the other parts of both male and female reproductive systems, are completely formed before birth, but only start functioning at puberty, between twelve and fifteen. Then the male sex hormone, called testosterone, begins to be produced in the body. The pituitary gland triggers this production. From then on sperm are produced by the body throughout life.

Sperm, which are miscroscopically small, are stored in a mass of tubing that is folded up and lies in a strip across the top of the testes. The sperm travel through a longer, thicker tube called the vas deferens, which leads up from under each testicle toward the seminal vesicles, located just under and in back of the bladder. Here the sperm mix with a milky fluid called semen.

The semen, and the millions of sperm it contains, travels through the urethra, a thin tube that runs out to the tip of the penis. The semen is ejaculated during intercourse.

How does the cell turn into a baby? When the mature female egg cell, or ovum, has been released from the ovary during ovulation, the ovum travels through the female's fallopian tube. If the male sperm meets and penetrates the female ovum in the tube fertilization takes place. The two cells merge into one, with a combined inheritance from both parents—one cell which, continuing on to the uterus, implanting itself, and growing there, will eventually become a new human being.

Does a baby start every time people mate? A baby is not formed unless a sperm meets and penetrates an ovum from the female. This does not always happen, since only one ovum is released each month. An ovum is capable of being fertilized for only forty-eight to seventy-two hours. However, since it is very difficult for anyone to know exactly when ovulation is occurring, it is necessary to use some method of birth control to prevent conception, if a baby is not desired.

Why does a baby look like its parents? A baby may look like his parents, or his great-grandparents, or his Uncle Henry. Both the male sperm and female ovum have a nucleus—a core or central point—which contains chromosomes. Chromosomes are made up of many thousands of tiny parts called genes,—and the particular combination of genes from each parent determines what characteristics will be inherited.

What causes twins? Cell division takes place within the covering, or shell, of the original cell. If the cell should split into two separate cells during the first division, two babies will develop. These are called identical twins, and will look exactly alike. Fraternal twins, which don't necessarily look alike and may even be boy and girl, are the result of two separate egg cells being fertilized, each by a different male sperm.

What causes birth defects? Young people at this age, fascinated as they are with the specifics of the reproductive process, are also curious about how and why birth defects occur. They have often seen telethons for various organizations collecting money for children born with such defects, and are both curious and anxious about how these occur. They can be told that only a very small percentage of infants are born with defects. Some are programmed into the genes and can be traced to a particular combination of hereditary qualities, such as in sickle-cell anemia, or Tay-Sachs disease, which can often be detected during pregnancy by genetic screening. What goes wrong can sometimes be traced to a factor in the prenatal environment—to a drug taken by the mother during pregnancy, such as thalidomide, or a virus that affects her at a crucial period during pregnancy, such as rubella, or German measles. Birth defects are due to a combination of hereditary and environmental influences, or damage during birth. Fortunately, great strides are being made in understanding these defects, and in treating them through better prenatal care, surgical intervention, and immunizations for rubella. During the preadolescent years, the growing interest in sex, however secretive it may be (and some of the interest may derive specifically from its undercover nature) is spurred by the glandular changes beginning to take place in the body. Since each individual matures at his or her own built-in pace, a twelve-year-old girl may have well-developed breasts, the rounded hips of a woman, and pubic hair, while her best friend of the same age may still look like nine year old—flat-chested with slim hips. Each wonders whether she is normal and needs to know that there is no set timetable for growth. Still, the flat-chested one may pester her mother for a training bra and spend her allowance on cosmetics and deodorants to keep up with her faster-developing friends.

Boys, too, while ostensibly preoccupied with the activities of their pals, will be anxiously looking for the signs of their coming manhood—enlarging genitals, hair on their bodies, even for the acne which will signify their emerging sexuality. Much anxiety and even fear about their mysterious physical and emotional changes can be allayed by knowledge about them and adequate preparation before they occur. Therefore, many schools, with the support of PTAs, are recognizing this with reality-geared sex-education programs in the early grades.

Since the period from nine to twelve is characterized for most youngsters by close ties to members of the same sex, it is not surprising that the sexual stirrings—which in a few short years will be "for real"—often express themselves in tentative sexual explorations with friends of the same sex. While this is more frequent among boys, whose physical roughhousing with other boys leads them into more body contact, it also occurs among girls. This may take the form of mutual masturbation, or oral and anal contacts. Many youngsters are secretly guilty and frightened by these activities, and unless they understand what is happening to them, may feel that they are becoming homosexual. While some few of them may always prefer sexual partners of the same sex, for most it is a phase which they will outgrow as they mature socially, emotionally, and physiologically. Pressuring such young people to begin dating members of the opposite sex is not the answer; they will find their own time if and when they are ready.

For some, the difference between accepting themselves as normal and being torn by conflicts about their sexual identity, which can leave longtime scars, will be the availability of a knowledgeable, accepting adult—whether parent, teacher or club leader—who can discuss their concerns with them in a natural, open way, and who can give them correct factual information and confirm the naturalness of this kind of sexual experimentation.

Parents often find the preadolescent, with his fierce loyalty to his friends and their codes of dress and behavior, so difficult to relate to that they give up in despair. Their own uncertainty is increased by the preadolescent's absolute certainty that he is greatly misunderstood and badly treated. Don't surrender to these feelings. These young people still need the guidance and support of parents. They are struggling to live up to two standards of behavior, the parents' and their peer group, which are bound to clash at many points. Most conflict arises when mothers and fathers feel that every new opinion of their child is a challenge to their own wisdom and must be fitted into their pattern or else stamped out. Learn to give a little. Don't hold on to authority for the sake of being the boss and at the expense of the young person's effort to widen his horizon and try his wings.

Parents hope that their youngster will learn without pain the hard lessons of growing up. This, somehow, does not seem possible to achieve, and children will be hurt as they grow. There are some situations, of course, in which the consequences of experimentation may be so destructive that the parent needs to be very firm and clear, as in the case of a child's taking dangerous drugs. Letting the child know the seriousness of the consequences, helping him get the facts, and considering the results of the options open to him in as objective a way as possible is a way of providing the support and guidance needed by him to resist the pressures from peers.

Your child's need to grow up and to be different from you by being himself is normal and necessary. He needs to test himself constantly against the values you hold, but if the parent has relinquished his own values out of uncertainty or fear, the child will feel lost, bewildered, and deserted.

V. The Adolescent Years: Ages Thirteen to Seventeen

How do physical changes affect the developing identity of young people? Normally, changes in boys are slow, and adjustments are gradual. During adolescence, however, physical changes are often drastic. The gangly teenage boy fills out; his hands and feet no longer seem impossibly large. His voice develops a deeper tone. He may start to shave or may grow a beard or moustache, depending on his life-style. His sexual organs mature and constantly react to visual, physical, and psychological stimuli.

The girl loses her sexless, little-girl slenderness, her hips widen, her breasts develop, her menstrual cycle settles into what will be her regular pattern. Both are biologically mature by age eighteen.

The way both boys and girls feel about their new bodily selves often reflects the way they feel about themselves generally. This is expressed in their concern, even preoccupation, with their physical appearance and how they dress. Some boys, unhappy with their physical development, may launch into a bodybuilding routine to develop their muscles into what they consider a suitably manly state. Girls may experiment with a variety of hairstyles, cosmetics—or no cosmetics at all. The appearance of skin blemishes, excess weight, or the non–appearance of breasts may be cause for tears, moodiness, or frantic applications of advertised cures. Boys may brood about what they consider the inadequate size of their sexual organs, and some members of both sexes may develop self-deprecatory attitudes about their supposed lack of physical desirability. Others couldn't care less about how they look—although sometimes this expressed lack of concern may conceal a sense of hopelessness about ever attaining some ideal standard. Still others are truly in rebellion against standards that they believe to be empty and meaningless, a rebellion expressed in a total rejection of the modes of dress, grooming, and even behavior of many of their peers.

Parents often find it difficult to know how to deal with the oversensitive feelings young people have about their appearance. They may have to guard against being too critical; it's hitting a sore spot. On the other hand, being reassuring may anger young people who feel that nobody understands them, or how difficult everything is for them, anyway. Probably the most parents can do is to listen for cues that ask for their help and offer whatever constructive suggestions they may have. They can certainly underscore the importance of the concept that it is not how one looks but what one is as a person that counts most heavily in the long run.

How do parents deal with young people whose clothes or hairstyles seem too bizaare? Parents insure a more flexible response from adolescents when they demonstrate flexibility themselves. A parent who issues a blanket statement to the effect that a particular mode of dress or hairstyle is *always* offensive is almost guaranteeing a similarly rigid attitude—in the opposite direction —from an adolescent.

It is always best to start with a recognition that everyone has the freedom to choose how he clothes himself before attempting to set limits on that freedom. When young people are allowed most of the time to dress as they wish, they are more likely to respond to parents' insistence on more conservative dress for important family or public occasions. Even then, this may be difficult or impossible for them because they may have too much at stake in the identity that their clothes give them.

Adolescents identify with others of their age, and the way in which they dress is a demonstration of their membership in a particular group. Parents have to consider that what they think is bizarre has to be reevaluated against the standards of the young. Adolescents have several reasons for resisting parents on this score: they value the acceptance of their peers, and they use their right to be different from their parents to establish some claim to independence.

At every developmental stage, the hallmark of increasing maturity is increasing independence. The progression from dependency to independence is evident in the gradual ability of children to walk, feed, and dress themselves without help. In older children, further independence is achieved as they learn to cross streets alone and travel unaccompanied for short and then longer distances.

Most parents find it easier to encourage physical rather than psychological independence. But even in families where children are encouraged to express their feelings and speak their minds, the rules seem to change in adolescence. More is at stake, mistakes can be more costly, and parents, formerly quite flexible, often become less able to permit their young to make their own decisions, and in some instances, become over–controlling. What often results is a battle of wills in which young people can't afford to lose their nearly won near-adult status. What they hear their parents saying in many of the conflicts about rights and privileges is that they are still children who should be dependent upon their parents' judgment. The only way to get around this impasse is to start with the understanding that the adolescent has to exercise his own judgment, but that parents have a responsibility to be involved in that process. Addressed on this level of shared responsibility, adolescents may respond more positively. As parents show their willingness to compromise, young people frequently do the same.

Some parents unwittingly keep their children locked in a relationship in which they are forever children. When these parents stand in the way of growing independence, adolescents have two alternatives—submit or rebel. The latter is the healthier alternative. However, adolescents may need help in seeing that freedom is also accompanied by responsibility.

There are a few ground rules that should be observed by parents when debating the issues of responsibility. First, they should steadfastly avoid a tendency to equate responsibility with economic self-sufficiency, an idea that results in arguments such as: "When you're old enough to earn a living, you can do as you please but until then. . . ." What one earns has little to do with his skill in exercising judgment; how he thinks does. (Nevertheless, parents can refuse to underwrite a plan with which they disagree on objective grounds.) Secondly, parents have to be willing to admit what they are feeling as well as what they are thinking: "I know you drive well enough to take the car but I feel anxious about the weather and would feel uncomfortable if you did." Or, if it happens to be true: "I don't think you drive well enough yet. I have to be sure." No youngster will be devastated by this hardheaded evaluation. But all of this—reasons, feelings, fears —has to be out in the open. Then a resolution can take place in which everyone gives a little, and a decision is made in the light of the needs of all of the people involved. Naturally, it's easier to talk about cars and clothing, but the same principles hold when sexuality is the issue.

Why are peers so important to adolescents? They need them. An adolescent's membership in a peer group is essential to his growth as an individual. It gives him status and social identity, and it provides opportunities for testing out new social skills. Adolescents do not always turn away from their parents and look exclusively to their peers for cues to acceptable social behavior. However, when they feel rejected or misunderstood, or when they feel unable to conform to their parents' expectations, they may become more vulnerable to the demands of the group or to pressures to experiment with, say, drugs or sex. In situations like these, parents have a tendency to set themselves up in hostile opposition to a group and all of its members. Some youngsters will be relieved and yield; others may be driven to align themselves more strongly with their friends.

If parents disagree with the standards of a peer group they need to make clear what their objections are and why they object. Adolescents have to learn to listen to what their parents think and what their peers think, and then to make their own choices.

How do adolescents find their own way? The critical question that the adolescent asks himself is, "Who am I?" by which he means, "What am I?" that is, "What kind of person am I?" "What are my special qualities?" "How are these qualities viewed by others?"

The answers to these questions embrace several facets of identity. The first of these is the biological fact of our sexual gender and the accident of birth into a particular family, community, and culture. The second is that which comes through continual interaction with others. We depend upon the reflected appraisals of others to tell us who and what we are. Finally, we have to answer to ourselves from an interior source that tells us—no matter how imperfectly—where we want to go and what we want to become. And we have to believe in the possibility that we have choices and the power to direct our own lives.

It takes more than a good body-image and affirmative relationships with others to build a stable sense of identity. Teenagers need a view of life in which there are options—not just one way to go. They also need to see themselves as capable of weighing the alternatives and making choices. What finally fuses the separate pieces of identity is the experience of making decisions and taking responsibility for their outcomes.

The age-old conflicts between adolescents and their parents are now intensified by pressures in a society that is changing at a rapid rate. Books, magazines, television, and films deal with subjects that used to be discussed—if at all—in private. Authority is no longer vested solely in parents. For example, some state legislatures are making it legal for young people to obtain medical treatment at age sixteen without parental consent, including contraceptive services, abortions, and treatment for venereal diseases. They are beginning to recognize young people's reluctance to discuss their sexual activities with their parents, and parents' unwillingness to face the need for such services for their young people.

Today's adolescents have options for sexual conduct that did not exist before, and seem able to engage in some form of sexual intimacy without the fear and guilt that agonized earlier generations. Our sexual codes are in a state of transition and many parents—as well as other adults who are in a position to influence the young—are uncertain about their ability to understand and interpret these new developments.

The first step in this process should be to confront the "myth of an abstinent past," as one researcher put it, and face more honestly the past as it actually was. Perhaps then parents can deal more realistically with the fact that adolescents today are not all that different from earlier generations—except that now they reach sexual maturity earlier and live in a less rigid and more open society.

Should teenagers go steady? Getting to know one person in a deeper and more sustained relationship is an important phase of emotional growth. Equally important is the development of social skills and a range of different responses that results from knowing many people. At every stage of their development, adolescents need to strike a balance between these two needs.

Teenagers go steady for a variety of reasons. Some boys and girls are not ready to cope with the pressures of dating a variety of people. They may not want to be involved in a competitive dating game, or they may shrink from exposure to sexual stimulation that they are not ready to handle. In the younger age groups, boys and girls will often choose "steadies" who do not make demands of them that they can't meet. Going steady for many of these youngsters is a form of mutual protection. A number of young adolescents go steady because it is the "in" thing to do. They may not be especially drawn to a particular boy or girl but need the social status of having a steady. Some of these arrangements may last a few weeks—or a few months. Going steady becomes a problem only for boys and girls who make their friendship an exclusive preoccupation that shuts out other friends.

Older adolescents may go steady for some of the same reasons. But if their development has proceeded normally, they will go steady because they have found a boy or girl who attracts them and whose company they prefer to others. It is this older group that concerns most parents, because of the recognition—open or suppressed—that sexual intimacy is a possibility in the developing relationship between sexually mature young people.

Should petting be discouraged? Petting is the term used to describe the physical contact—short of intercourse—that results in sexual arousal and sometimes an orgasm. It has been part of the repertory of human sexual responses for thousands of years and is common to many different kinds of cultures. It appears to be so deeply ingrained in human behavior that even the most active discouragement of its practice is unlikely to be effective. Social or parental taboos against petting appear to produce guilt feelings rather than a change in behavior.

In order to discourage petting, parents would have to align themselves with a position in which not only premarital intercourse but any form of sexual expression is prohibited before marriage. Except in a rigidly controlled social environment, this would be a very difficult position for parents to maintain. Nevertheless, many parents are worried about the ways in which petting may lead to sexual intercourse.

One of the reasons why petting *does* often lead to intercourse is that young people are so uninformed about the nature of sexual response in the male and female and are easy prey for the sexual myths that circulate among their peers. Thus many girls are pressured into permitting sexual intercourse before they are ready to commit themselves that fully, by boys who—possibly believing it themselves—think it will make them "crazy" if they pet to orgasm without intercourse. This, of course, is only one of a number of come-ons.

Parents—or those who serve as guides to the young—do have the responsibility of informing young people that boys are more easily aroused than girls, and once aroused, find it difficult to restrain their sexual impulse to achieve orgasm. Girls, usually slower to arousal, can also tolerate much more stimulation without the same urgency for orgasm. Both need to know that petting to orgasm is an alternative to sexual intercourse, recognizing also that sperm deposited near the vagina can sometimes, if rarely, cause pregnancy.

Prepared with correct information about how boys function and an opportunity to consider the risks they run when they permit themselves to engage in petting (or when they seduce a boy into this activity), girls may indeed prefer the option of saying no—an option many of them don't even know they have. Many young girls feel obligated to "pay" for the privilege of being taken to a movie or dance—a sorry commentary on the value system they have absorbed. But a girl needs a strong sense of her own worth as a person—a person who is worthwhile to be with, whether she is ready for a sexual encounter or not—to be able to deal with an importunate male.

Of course many girls, even very young girls, are openly provocative, or coy and seductive, in both dress and manner but are not always ready for the sexual response they arouse. Girls are apt to be more interested in the "romantic" aspects of being admired and desired; boys are usually happy to oblige (although there are some who are definitely frightened off by these challenges), and will declare their love and affection most readily to achieve the goal of sexual release. Unless a girl understands this, she may get emotionally bruised by what she took to be a real attachment.

Yet for many adolescents, petting does not inevitably lead to sexual intercourse. Some engage in oral-genital contacts because they have so often been warned about the possible negative results of intercourse. There is evidence, in fact, that the highest incidence of premarital intercourse has occurred in groups in which petting is minimal. When petting results in satisfaction and the release of sexual tension, some adolescents do not have the need to go on to sexual intercourse, and this may indeed enable them to remain virgins if they prefer to do so.

Does information about contraception encourage adolescents to engage in sexual intercourse? There is no evidence to support the idea that birth-control information increases the likelihood that adolescents will engage in sexual intercourse. The decision—or the impulse—to engage in sexual activity is based upon many factors, and knowing about contraception seems to be a secondary consideration. When strong sexual drives or compelling emotional reasons result in sexual intimacy, the fear of pregnancy, even when it is very strong, seems to be pushed into the background.

According to a number of careful studies, many sexually active young people are either ignorant or seriously misinformed about birth-control methods. Some of them, for example, believe that pregnancy cannot result from the first sexual experience or cannot happen unless one is married. Others think that Saran Wrap is as effective as a condom or that douching with Seven-Up or other carbonated beverages prevents conception. Still others risk pregnancy because they think they can predict their "safe period"—an idea that grows out of faulty sex education or half-understood information about the menstrual cycle. Much of this misinformation comes from listening to their peers, who are equally misinformed. In the absence of sound sex education, myths like these continue to be passed on as facts.

Parents and teachers have the responsibility of correcting the erroneous information that many adolescents already have about birth-control methods and providing the correct information. Knowledge about contraception by itself neither prevents nor encourages sexual intercourse. The open discussion of the options that are available to individuals who wish to prevent an unwanted pregnancy, however, may have the effect of impressing young people with the responsibilities that accompany sexually active behavior. The need is for more education, not less.

Nevertheless, parents are often reluctant to talk about contraception with adolescents, feeling that by so doing they will be encouraging or condoning sexual activity. Moreover, after the early years of adolescence, young people, whether sexually active or not, rarely come to their parents for such information. They may anticipate a response such as, "What do you need that information for?"—a question they usually prefer not to answer, fearing they will be "hassled" if they do. Nevertheless, few parents, faced with the alternative of having a young person risk pregnancy by being sexually active without using adequate contraception, would deny her access to contraceptive services. Since the ultimate choice of being sexually active or not is up to the young person and not the parent, the giving of information should be perceived as providing the means for making an informed choice.

What are the currently available contraceptive methods? Not having intercourse is still the only guaranteed way to prevent pregnancy, and young people need to know that. It is one of the options open to them, and some of them choose it.

If the decision is to be sexually active, but to take the precautions necessary to prevent conception, the adolescent must be familiar with the methods that work (as well as those that don't) and choose the one most suited to his or her life-style, personal tastes, and physical capacity to utilize. Most of the methods that work best must be medically prescribed (preferably by a gynecologist), and some, such as the birth-control pill, should be medically supervised as well.

The most effective method is the birth-control pill, which consists of two chemicals, estrogen and progesterone, basically the same as the hormones a woman's own body makes to stop release of egg cells during pregnancy. (Actually there are a variety of pills of varying dosages, suitable for individual needs.)

Going on the "Pill" means going on a schedule: One pill every day for a set number of days every month—twenty, twenty-one, or twenty-eight depending on the kind of pill. It is the day-by-day action of the whole series, not any one pill, that gives the protection, by keeping the body from releasing its monthly egg cell. With no egg to meet, there's no possible chance of an egg-sperm meeting, therefore no chance of pregnancy.

While there are risks involved in taking the pill, as there are with any drug, they are known to be minimal if the pill is prescribed by a physician who takes a medical history, screens out all candidates who suffer from certain physical conditions, and then monitors the patient regularly. She is required to return periodically for checkups and to report any side effects. (Such side effects as slight nausea the first few months and shorter menstrual periods with less flow are normal.) The pill can also be obtained at Planned Parenthood clinics, most of which have special services for young people.

Another effective method which must be medically prescribed is the diaphragm (always used in conjunction with spermicidal cream or jelly). The diaphragm is a thin rubber shield that is smeared with special cream or jelly, and placed deep inside the vagina, where it fits snugly over the cervix, or entrance to the uterus. That is why it must be fitted by a physician, as each woman is different. Any sperm entering the vagina on its way to meet the egg is blocked two ways: physically by the diaphragm and chemically by the spermicidal cream or jelly, which kills sperm. It must be used every time intercourse takes place according to the instructions given by the physician. It has no side effects.

The third effective method is the IUD, or intrauterine device, meaning it goes inside the uterus. It must be inserted by a specially trained physician and removed by him when it is no longer needed. Once in place it can remain unfelt for months or years. Nothing more needs to be done about birth control, except that the woman needs to feel for the tiny strings that let her know that the IUD is in place. There are a number of theories about how the IUD works, but no one knows exactly. Some women's bodies will not tolerate it, and the uterus pushes the IUD out. Some women have been known to get pregnant with the IUD in place. However, newer varieties of IUDs are proving more effective and easier to retain. ·

A very good method, particularly for young people who may hesitate to seek medically prescribed methods, is the condom, which is used by the male in conjunction with the spermicidal cream, jelly, or foam, used by the female.

The condom (or rubber, safety, prophylactic, shin, sheath, bag) can be purchased at any drugstore. Made of strong but thin rubber, it fits over the penis and catches and holds the semen when it is released, so no sperm get into the vagina. An additional advantage of the condom is that it provides some protection against venereal disease. However, it must be put on properly (after the penis is erect but before it gets near the vagina, as sperm can be released before ejaculation), and space must be left at the tip to accommodate the semen when it is ejaculated. The condom should be held at the part nearest the body when the penis relaxes so it won't slip off before or during withdrawal.

Just in case the condom should break (which happens rarely, but just in case), additional protection is provided if the female uses spermicidal vaginal foam, cream, or jelly (not feminine hygiene products.) Spermicidal creams such as vaginal foaming tablets or suppositories can be purchased at the drugstore. They work by setting up a chemical roadblock in the vagina, and come with special applicators that measure the proper amount and help to get it in the right place.

Foams, creams, and jellies must be used every time sexual inter-course occurs, and must be applied not more than half an hour before coitus takes place.

Withdrawal (or "getting out in time"), while as old as man, is very chancy, as some semen is often released before ejaculation.

The rhythm method, which relies on abstaining from inter-course during a woman's fertile period, requires medical super-vision to work out the woman's supposed time of ovulation and very careful charting of the menstrual cycle. It is useful only for very highly motivated couples.

Planned Parenthood clinics throughout the country provide information about birth-control methods, as well as services.

Why do girls continue to become pregnant when contraceptives are effective and available? In spite of the greater effectiveness and availability of contraceptives, a number of adolescent girls become pregnant either because they are ignorant about birth-control methods or use them incorrectly (like the girls who "pop" a pill when going on a date, believing that one birth-control pill will give them protection), or they use methods that give them no protection or involve a high degree of risk, such as products advertised for "feminine hygiene" which suggest that they are contraceptives but actually aren't.

While some teenage pregnancies are the result of accident or carelessness, others are motivated—knowingly or unknowingly—by a girl's desire to coerce a boy into marriage or to bolster a shaky identity. Insecure girls may view pregnancy as a way of demonstrating that they are sexually desirable or have achieved the status of adults. For those who have been unsuccessful in developing an identity through other channels, this may be perceived as an option. For them, motherhood, with or without marriage, provides an instant identity. Other girls may be motivated to become pregnant to spite their parents. Pregnancy for them becomes a means of demonstrating their rebellion against family and society.

Many experts in the field believe that contraceptive information and services alone cannot be expected to prevent teenage pregnancies because so many of our traditional cultural values actually predispose girls to become pregnant. One of these is the idea of feminine passivity, which makes girls feel more comfortable if they are—or pretend to be—seduced or coerced into sexual activity. Another is the romantic idea in which sexual activity is valid only when it is impulsive or spontaneous. Thinking about or using contraceptives introduces a note of premeditation that violates these values. There are indications that girls who are brought up to believe that marriage and motherhood are the only worthwhile goals for women may be more vulnerable to unwanted pregnancies. Girls who have career objectives, on the other hand, seem to be more inclined to avoid pregnancy and to postpone marriage.

Parents sometimes need to be reminded that adolescent boys as well as girls need and want correct information about male and female sexual functioning, about their own role and responsibility in sexual activity and reproduction. A boy, too, needs to know that he can be emotionally damaged by sexual involvements that he is not ready for, and that he too can have his life goals short–circuited by impregnating a girl before he is ready to be a father.

A good omen for the future is the increasing mutuality of decision-making between boys and girls about sexual activity, with boys more frequently taking responsibility for use of the male contraceptive—the condom—and for accompanying their girls to a birth-control clinic for contraceptive education and services.

What about abortion? Abortion, the surgical procedure performed to put an end to a pregnancy, is now legally available to any woman who, with medical approval, makes a decision to have one within the first three months of pregnancy.

Since abortion was illegal in this country from the late nineteenth century until the United States Supreme Court ruled it a personal right in January 1973, and since it has been opposed by some religious groups on various theological and moral grounds, it retains a degree of unacceptability in some quarters. Moreover, a deeply ingrained respect for the value of human life, even from its earliest inception, makes it difficult for many people to come to terms with abortion as a desirable procedure. Before it became legal, however, it is estimated that at least one million illegal abortions were performed in this country each year, creating serious medical risks for those who preferred to take this course rather than to carry an unwanted pregnancy to term.

However each individual may feel about it, it is now a woman's right. Certain limitations set by medical authorities in the various states are designed to protect her health.

It is important for parents and young people to know that abortion within the first three months of pregnancy is a simple medical procedure; after this period it is more complicated, more costly, and less safe. Should an adolescent girl become pregnant, she should have an opportunity to consider all the options open to her: carrying the pregnancy to term and have the baby, keeping it herself, giving it up for adoption, or having an abortion. Some young people, with or without parental pressure, marry to give the baby a name and a home; many such marriages do not last but can be traumatic and long lasting in their ill effects. According to statistics, over half of all teenage marriages are performed under these conditions.

Adoption agencies across the country operate homes for girls who choose to have their babies. The girl lives in a special home during her pregnancy, after which she may decide to keep the child, place it in foster care, or give it up for adoption. However, with the opportunity to remain in school despite pregnancy, many girls are opting to stay at home, continue with their education, and keep babies with help from their families.

Those girls, married or unmarried, who choose to have an abortion should receive a simple pregnancy test as soon as possible, which is about two weeks after the date of the first missed menstrual period. If the test is positive, it must be confirmed by a physician (preferably a gynecologist) who will determine the exact stage of the pregnancy. If her own physician is not prepared to perform the abortion for her, he should refer her to an appropriate and qualified resource.

The first-trimester abortion is usually performed by vacuum aspiration, a method whereby a plastic tube (about the size of a pencil) that is attached to a suction pump is introduced into the vagina. The suction pump then draws out the embryo. This procedure is usually performed under local anesthesia, in a medically approved outpatient facility or hospital, and takes fifteen to twenty minutes.

The other method utilized is called a D and C (dilation and curettage), in which the contents of the uterus are removed by scraping with an instrument known as a curette. General anesthesia is more usual with D and C. Some hospitals prefer that the girl stay the night before, and some prefer she stay the night after as well.

Between the thirteenth and sixteenth week of pregnancy, abortions are usually not performed. Most physicians feel it is too late for a safe suction or D and C to be performed, and the conditions are not optimal for performing other methods which should be done later in the pregnancy.

Between the sixteenth and twentieth weeks of pregnancy, a method known as the saline procedure is used. This consists of removing some of the fluid in the uterus and replacing it with a concentrated mixture of salt and water. This brings on labor contractions some twelve to forty-eight hours later, and the fetus is expelled. This procedure is usually performed in a hospital, under local anesthesia. Still another procedure used, although very rarely, is the hysterotomy, a mini-ceasarean section, that requires cutting into the abdomen and uterus. This is major surgery, with its attendant greater risks and costs.

Obviously, an early abortion is preferable to later abortion procedures. If a young person is able to acknowledge her sexual activity and face the possibility of pregnancy honestly, she will be able to take steps in time to get an early abortion if that is her choice.

Equally apparent is the desirability of adequate sex education, knowledge about one's choices in opting for sexual activity or not, and adequate information about contraception to avoid the possibility of the need for an abortion.

An adolescent's education for responsible sexuality, whether provided by parents or other knowledgeable adults, must include information about male and female anatomy and modes of sexual response, correct and adequate information about contraception, and enlightened recognition of the emotional as well as physical needs that determine sexual behavior. Young people are then familiar with the options open for them to make their own choices—choices, however, that will be influenced by the values with which they have been reared and by the examples which their families have provided all along.

What about venereal diseases? In recent years there has been a growing epidemic of venereal diseases—syphilis and gonorrhea—

among young people. Whether this reflects a general increase in sexual activity among the teenage population, or a greater willingness to go for treatment, thus increasing the statistics on reported cases, the fact is that syphilis is a major killer among the communicable diseases and the incidence of gonorrhea is particularly high among those twenty-five years of age and under. Since most schools provide information in health-education classes about the grave dangers of these diseases, it is obvious that fear of infection, like fear of pregnancy, is not a deterrent to sexual activity. Perhaps the same "magical" thinking of it-can't-happen-to-me operates in both instances. And perhaps lack of correct information on the part of both parents and young people, and their unwillingness to talk about anything related to sex, is responsible in part for the rapid increase in the incidence of these dangerous diseases. For syphilis and gonorrhea can only be caught through sexual contact with individuals of the same or opposite sex. The germs that cause these diseases cannot live outside the human body for more than a few seconds, so they cannot be caught from toilet seats or dirty drinking glasses.

What are the symptoms? Syphilis (pox, lues, bad blood, siff, haircut, old Joe) affects men and women in very much the same way. The syphilis germ enters the body through the skin in or around the genitals or mouth. The first sign may be a sore which shows up in ten to ninety days, usually at the place where the germ enters the body. It may appear though, on the finger or even the breast. When a person has such a sore, or chancre, he or she is said to have syphilis in its primary stage. Sometimes the chancre doesn't show up at all, or it may be so small as to go unnoticed. Or it may be hidden deep inside a woman's sex organs where it cannot be seen. At any rate, it doesn't hurt.

The chancre may look like a pimple, blister, or open sore; if it is apparent, it is very dangerous to others, since it is full of germs. Soon after the appearance of this sore, the germs begin to spread through the body. At this stage a blood test will show positive. Whether the person is treated or not, the sore will go away, but the germs are still inside the body, increasing in number and spreading throughout.

From three to six weeks later a rash may appear on the body or on hands and feet; sores may appear in the mouth; a sore throat, fever, or headache may develop; hair may fall out in patches. This is called the secondary stage and may resemble many other diseases. Unless a person has a blood test, he may not realize he has it. These secondary symptoms will also disappear without any treatment, but by this time the disease may begin to attack the heart, brain, and spinal cord. The individual may feel normal and healthy for many years, but eventually he will become blind, insane, or crippled in other ways, or will die of syphilitic heart disease.

If a woman has syphilis while pregnant, she can pass the disease on to her baby; the baby may be born prematurely or be stillborn. Or it may be born with hidden syphilis, which can later cause it to become blind, deaf, paralyzed, or insane, or to die. Every expectant mother should have a blood test; if she is treated before her fifth month of pregnancy, her child will be protected from this disease.

Gonorrhea is caused by a different germ than syphilis but is also caught by sexual contact. It is much more prevalent and contagious than syphilis, but it is harder to diagnose, particularly in women, since four out of five women may show no symptoms. One out of five men may show no symptoms, though usual symptoms are a painful burning sensation during urination and a messy yellow-white discharge from the penis. Since gonorrhea is apt to have fewer or no symptoms, if a person has been exposed the only sure method of diagnosis is to have a doctor take a smear, which he can examine under a microscope or send to a laboratory for testing.

Gonorrhea appears three to five days after contact with an infected person, and without treatment can damage the sperm ducts of the male, or fallopian tubes of the female, thus affecting fertility. It can also lead to a crippling form of arthritis, meningitis, or heart disease.

Many states have passed special laws enabling young people to go for treatment to doctors, or public health clinics without obtaining the consent of their parents.

While syphilis and gonorrhea have different symptoms, and are diagnosed in different ways, they must both be diagnosed early. They are treatable by injections of penicillin (or other drugs if there is an allergy to penicillin). Both can be caught again—even if they have been diagnosed, treated, and cured—by contact with an infected person.

What is homosexuality?

Homosexuality, as distinguished from *homosexual behavior,* is the preference for a person of the same gender as a partner in sexual and emotional relationships. It is, in a sense, a life-style, since sexual and emotional attraction to members of the same sex is a basic part of the personality structure of homosexual individuals, whether or not it is expressed in overt acts.

Homosexual behavior is engaged in by a large number of people, most of whom are not homosexuals. The studies by Kinsey and other recent researchers show that more than one-third of American males have participated in homosexual behavior, to the point of orgasm, at least once in their postadolescent lives, and some people, known as bisexuals are able to enjoy sexual and emotional relationships with both sexes. Only about 5 percent of American males and 2 percent of American females are exclusively homosexual throughout their lives.

We know too little about the causes of homosexuality, or for that matter, of heterosexuality, to state with any assurance what they are. On the basis of what little is known, it appears that early environmental factors—such as the parents' relationship to each other, their preferences for male and female children, and the kind of relationship each develops with the child—play an important role in the development of both the individual's sexual orientation, as hetero-, bi-, or homosexual, and of his or her sexual identity as a man or a woman.

A homosexual orientation does not mean the individual is something less than a man or less than a woman. Homosexual males, as with heterosexual males, define themselves as men; homosexual females (sometimes known as lesbians), as with heterosexual females, define themselves as women. For example, homosexual individuals usually cannot be identified by their appearance. Gentle, artistic, or feminine-looking boys and men are not necessarily homosexual, nor are aggressive or masculine-looking girls and women. Indeed, the opposite is just as often the case —some great male athletes, recognized as the epitome of masculinity, are homosexuals, as are many feminine women, who may even be mothers but who prefer a female sexual partner.

Homosexuals come in all shapes and sizes, from all religious, ethnic, and racial groups, and all socio–economic levels, from the Wall Street banker to the hard hat. The only certain criterion for homosexuality is the sexual preference of the individual for members of his or her own gender.

In many cultures homosexuality was an accepted life-style for some segments of society. This is not so in the modern Western societies, where homosexuality (and homosexual behavior) has been condemned as a crime, a sin, or a sign of serious psychological maladjustment.

More recently, the social and moral climate has changed dramatically with regard to homosexuality and homosexual acts between consenting adults. An increasing number of leading psychiatrists and other health professionals support the view that homosexuality is a valid variant life-style, and that therapy for troubled individuals should attempt to increase the individual's comfort with himself or herself as a sexual person, whether heterosexual or homosexual, and should be more concerned with improving the quality of relationships rather than with trying—rarely effectively, no matter how highly motivated the individual may be for change—to force a different sexual orientation. Most religious denominations are re–examining their traditional views of homosexuality, defining homosexuals as "persons of sacred worth" or "sinners as we all are sinners."

Because of society's attitudes about homosexuality, many homosexuals, heretofore fearful of social ostracism, of losing their jobs, of being arrested, have begun to identify themselves publicly and to organize in political and social groups that speak out against the discrimination, harassment, and deprivation of certain of their civil rights that they face in their daily lives. These groups challenge the view that homosexuals are sick, and demand that homosexuals, or "gays," be as free as heterosexuals are to live their own lives, subject to the same social controls and to be treated by the "straight" society as any other citizens, different from their peers only by virtue of their sexual preferences.

By the time a child has reached adolescence, his or her sexual orientation, whether heterosexual or homosexual, is well established, even though this may not declare itself until adult life. But during preadolescence and the early adolescent years, both boys and girls often experiment sexually with friends of their own sex, and some become concerned as to whether or not they might be homosexuals. Should they seek counsel and advice from their parents, they usually can be assured that this is only a phase of their development. Whether or not they will be able to communicate with their parents about these matters will depend on the degree of trust that exists and the openness and respect with which their previous sex questions have been handled.

By eighteen or nineteen years of age, the individual's concerns may be more troubling or anxiety producing. In such cases professional guidance or counseling may help these young people to come to terms with themselves as to who they really are.

Parents who discover that their child is a homosexual should realize that he or she is the same child they have loved and cherished since birth, and that he or she has not suddenly become a different person. They should accept their homosexual child as he or she is, and offer the same love and emotional support that they give their other children.

What attitude can a parent reasonably assume about premarital intercourse? It is easier for parents to be open-minded with each other and with their young people when they are willing to acknowledge that there are no simple answers of right and wrong in dealing with the complex issues of sexual morality. What may be right for one person may be questionable for another, depending on many circumstances. Since people tend to become rigid and righteous in their attitudes when they are anxious and uncertain, both parents and young people will need to be very honest with themselves and each other in recognizing all the factors that must be considered in deciding such issues. In the end, people must do what feels right for them. It is the basis on which they make their decisions that becomes important.

There are times when feelings and reality collide, producing apparent contradictions. One example of this is the situation in which older adolescents bring home as a house guest a friend with whom they are engaged in a sexually intimate relationship. Having given their tacit approval to the relationship, parents nevertheless feel uncomfortable about making arrangements for the couple to share the same room. This may seem inconsistent—and it is—and to young people may seem to be hypocritical. Nevertheless, it is legitimate for parents to say in effect "We are more comfortable with this traditional arrangement in our own home —elsewhere you are free to live as you wish."

There is a general assumption that premarital intercourse is more widespread than it used to be, at least as it relates to young women. This is borne out by competent research. But it is also true that there is more openness, honesty, and acceptance about sexual matters today. The double standard of sexual morality that existed in the past, when it was more or less expected that young men would "sow their wild oats" before marriage (usually with prostitutes or women who were considered their social inferiors) has given way to sexual relationships between social equals, with emphasis on affectional bonds and a mutuality of interests. More young people of both sexes are apparently viewing premarital intercourse as an option rather than a prohibition. It is something they may or may not do but their reasons for deciding one way or the other are based on personal considerations and not on fear of exposure or social censure.

These days many young people are confronted with pressures to lose their virginity rather than to keep it. Sometimes the pressure comes from peers: from boys who are inclined to see intercourse as a rite of initiation into maturity or from girls who may be uncomfortable about their own sexual experiences and need the reassurance that it is acceptable by recruiting other girls to their ranks. Sometimes the pressure comes from a boy who wants a girl to prove that she really cares for him—as if caring is invalid without sexual expression—or from a girl who is overly aggressive or possessive.

Young people need opportunities to experience support from others to postpone a sexual experience for which they feel they are not ready. They also need to be sensitized to the ways in which sexual needs are exploited for non–sexual purposes—for power, control, submission, and acceptance—and to develop self-awareness and awareness of the purposes of others. To allow oneself to be used selfishly can be emotionally eroding and destructive.

Fortunately, society has moved away from the puritanical idea that sex outside of marriage is always bad. It would be equally unfortunate if we were to delude ourselves that it is always good.

As parents, what we want to give our children most of all is the capacity to love. This we do first by loving them and by responding to their love for us. Later we must be ready to stand aside when they begin to turn their interest and affection to others outside the family, and finally to their chosen partner. If we can show by our own example that love is based on mutual respect, whether it is expressed sexually or in another manner, we will have done much to point the way toward leading a rewarding and self-fulfilling life.

VI. If You Need Help

If your child's problems are too complex for you to handle alone, you can often get help from trained people in your community. Such people usually can be found in the guidance department of the school, in a family-service agency, a child-guidance clinic or a public health center. If you do not know about such services, the Health and Welfare Council in your community can give you information and suggest sources of help. Or you might want to talk to your own physician or religious adviser, or to a psychiatrist.

If you have no local source of information, write to the Family Service Association of America, 44 East Twenty-third Street, New York, New York 10010, or Planned Parenthood Federation of America, 810 Seventh Avenue, New York, New York 10019.

Selected Readings for Parents, Children, and Young People

Since sexual development is part of a child's total growth, several books in the following adult reading list deal with child development in general. Other pamphlets range from family planning to material on children from infancy.

In selecting a book to be shared with children, read it first to check its appropriateness for the individual child and your situation. It might also offer further guidance in dealing with the questions you are being asked. While books alone cannot substitute for the essential personal communication between adults and children about the meaning of being male or female, they frequently can be of special help and support.

Some young people seem to enjoy reading books about human growth, yet others appear to dislike them. A child's attitude may change, however, depending on his inner need at a given moment. Because every child matures at a different rate, the decision about when to share a book will depend on your best judgment as to when he seems ready for it. The age groupings are merely suggested.

Suggested Reading for Parents and Other Adults

Adolescent Sexuality in Contemporary America, Robert C. Sorenson. World Publishing, 1973 ($20.00).

    Study of adolescents' attitudes and behavior.

The Future of Marriage, Jessie Bernard. World Publishing, 1972 ($9.95).

    In a provocative and philosophical book, Dr. Bernard examines what marriage does for and to men and women today, and the multiplicity of options that she thinks will be open to both sexes in the future. Her in-depth exploration of the human needs underlying the changing institution of marriage will interest thoughtful parents.

Childhood and Adolescence: A Psychology of the Growing Person, L. Joseph Stone and Joseph Church. 3rd ed., Random House, 1973 ($10.95).

    An outstanding text on child development, emphasizing the dynamic process of growth toward maturity, and written with empathy for both children and parents. This edition takes into account newer research dealing with the prenatal newborn, and infancy periods, and later cognitive development.

Caring for Your Disabled Child, Benjamin M. Spock, M.D. and Marion O. Lerrigo. Macmillan, 1965 ($4.95).

Contains suggestions on ways to guide a physically, mentally, or emotionally handicapped child in sexual and social adjustment, and on possible marriage problems.

Concerns of Parents About Sex Education, The Reverend Thomas E. Brown. SIECUS, 1971 ($.50).

Written in a question-discussion format, this SIECUS study guide identifies common situations parents experience in teaching their children about sexuality. Available by mail from 1855 Broadway, New York, New York 10025.

Heredity in Humans, Amram Sheinfeld. Rev. ed., illus., J. B. Lippincott, 1972 ($6.95).

This storehouse of information about heredity is a classic reference book. The writing is nontechnical, interesting, and easy reading for the layman.

Conception, Birth, and Contraception: A Visual Presentation, Robert Demarest and John J. Sciarra, M.D.. McGraw-Hill, 1969 ($8.95).

Although there is no attempt here to deal with the emotional aspects of sex and reproduction, this book is an excellent pictorial scientific presentation of the subject.

Love, Sex, and Being Human, Paul Bohannon. Doubleday, 1969 (paper, $1.45).

This brief volume contains an excellent presentation of the physiological and emotional aspects of sexual growth, and the moral and ethical dilemmas that face the sexually mature person.

Sex and Your Teenager, Eda LeShan. David McKay, 1969 ($5.95)

An open-ended and liberal guide for parents in tune with the needs and attitudes of today's young people.

Sex in the Adolescent Years: New Directions in Guiding and Teaching Youth, ed. by Isadore Rubin and Lester A. Kirkendall. Association Press, 1968 ($4.95).

This realistic exploration of many areas of sex education offers sound approaches for educators and parents. It calls for a willingness on the part of the older generation to face social reality and changes that inevitably occur between generations, particularly in a dynamic society such as ours.

Analysis of Human Sexual Response, ed. by Ruth and Edward Brecher. New American Library, 1966 (paper, $1.25).

A husband-wife team of science writers skillfully interprets findings of the Masters-Johnson sex research. This book should resolving longstanding controversies about the nature of the female orgasm and the effects of sex during pregnancy. It also covers other important medical and emotional aspects of human sexuality. It includes chapters by well-known professional persons on related studies (some anthropological), the history of sex research, and a critique of the puzzling problems of taste and values that such research poses.

The Responsive Parent: Meeting the Realities of Parenthood Today, Mary B. Hoover. Parents Magazine Press, 1972 ($5.95).

A fully rounded picture of life with growing children and developing parents.

Who Shall Live: Man's Control over Birth and Death, American Friends Service Committee. Hill and Wang, 1970 ($3.95).

Discuss many complex and emotional issues—the population explosion, abortion, definition of death, and the quality of life. Index and bibliography.

Sexuality and Man, compiled and ed. by SIECUS. Scribner's, 1970 ($6.95).

A collection of papers, mostly issued previously as SIECUS study guides, covering assorted topics such as psychosexual development throughout the life cycle, premarital sexual standards, masturbation, and child molestation.

V.D.: The ABC's, John W. Grover and Richard Grace. Prentice-Hall, 1971 (paper, $2.95).

An excellent, simply written, nonjudgmental coverage of all the facts about venereal diseases, their symptoms, treatment, and prevalence.

The Magic Years, Selma H. Fraiberg. Scribner's, 1959 (paper, $2.45).
This exceptionally fine book about the child's first five years includes a noteworthy section, "Education for Love," making a distinction between sex instruction and the total responsibility of sex education.

For Children Five to Nine

A Baby is Born: The Story of How Life Begins, Milton I. Levine and Jean Seligmann. Rev. ed., Golden Press, 1962 (paper, $1.00).
This graphically illustrated book describes the events that contribute to the beginning of life and presents physiological facts in the order in which children's questions usually arise.

How Babies Are Made, Andrew C. Andry and Steven Schepp. Time-Life Books, 1968 ($3.95).
The story of reproduction in plants, animals, and humans is told through the use of color photographs of paper sculptures. Factually accurate and simple enough to be understood by the youngest age group.

The Story of A Baby, Marie Ets. Rev. Ed., Viking Press, 1969 ($3.75).
To be read aloud to the younger child, this book presents a detailed treatment of the fertilization and gestation processes with clear drawings.

The Wonderful Story of How You Were Born, Sidonie Matsner Gruenberg. Rev. ed., Doubleday, 1970 ($3.95).
Writing as a grandmother telling a story, an authority on child development explains the facts of conception, birth, and growth. The first part will help answer a young child's questions; the second part offers more detail for older children.

For Children Nine to Twelve

Facts About Sex: A Basic Guide, Sol Gordon, Ph.D. John Day
Co., 1970 (paper, $1.90)
   Written at a sixth-grade reading-comprehension level, this
book was originally published for retarded adolescents. It presents the facts of life in a brief and frank language that includes terms likely to be familiar to young people. The book
is well illustrated and contains a list of references.

How Life Begins, Jules Power. Simon and Shuster, 1965 ($4.95).
   A unity of text, photographs, and drawings that illuminate
with taste the subject of where babies come from and how
they develop.

Love and Sex and Growing Up, Eric W. Johnson and Corrine B.
Johnson. J. B. Lippincott, 1970 ($3.95).
   A book for preadolescents that covers a broad range of
topics: differing family patterns and the kinds of individuals
each produces; divorce; being widowed; choosing not to marry;
human growth and development; plant and animal reproduction. Helps a young person to think about what being a man
or a woman means in today's world.

For Later Teens

Sex: Telling It Straight, Eric W. Johnson. J. B. Lippincott, 1970
($3.95).
   A simple but honest treatment of those topics in human sexuality of greatest concern to adolescents. This book is written
for teenage slow readers, especially those within a ghetto environment, and presents positive views on sex without preach-
ing or moralizing.

Love and Sex in Plain Language, Eric W. Johnson. J. B. Lippincott, 1973 ($4.95).
   The author of *How to Live Through Junior High School*
and *Love and Sex in Plain Language* has written a book that

is simple enough for young adolescents and factually complete enough for older ones. He puts the decision of when and how to use one's sexual powers squarely up to the individual. Parents may also find the book useful.

Boys and Sex, Wardell P. Pomeroy, Ph.D. Delacorte Press, 1968 ($4.50).

A sexual guide for teenage boys written in a straightforward, objective, and nonjudgmental way, using language that is easily understood.

Girls and Sex, Wardell B. Pomeroy, Ph.D. Delacorte Press, 1969 ($4.50).

As in his earlier book, *Boys and Sex,* Wardell Pomeroy presents his views in an open way without moralizing and with no attempt to discourage teenage girls from engaging in sexual activities if they are psychologically ready.

Commonsense Sex, Ronald M. Mazur. Beacon Press, 1968 ($3.95)

Aimed at unmarried individuals, this book covers such sensitive subjects as masturbation, contraception, premarital intercourse, mutual masturbation, and homosexuality. The book is based on the premise that sex is a positive aspect of human personality and concludes with a suggestion of a liberal religious framework for decision making.

Growing Up with Sex, Richard F. Hettlinger. Seabury Press, 1971 (paper, $2.25).

Relegating anatomical and reproductive facts to a series of appendices, the author thoroughly describes sexual behavior without moralizing but with respect for more traditional mores.

Sex Before Twenty: New Answers for Youth, Helen F. Southard. Rev. ed., E. P. Dutton, 1971 ($4.50).

In this book, teenagers are encouraged to take responsibility for themselves in discovering their full role as sexual persons. The discussion of male and female roles in this edition shows the influence of both male and female liberation.

Why Wait Till Marriage, Evelyn M. Duvall. Association Press, 1968 (paper, $.75).

Written within a broadly religious framework, this book deals one by one with arguments favoring premarital intercourse. Not only intended for adolescents, it will give youth leaders and parents some insights into today's changing sex patterns.

For Young Adults

The Student Guide to Sex on Campus, Student Committee on Human Sexuality, Yale University. New American Library, 1970 (pap., $1.00).

In addition to offering excellent information on contraceptives, abortion, sterilization, venereal disease, and male and female sexual anatomy, this book deals with other questions about sexuality that young people are asking today.

Birth Control: Methods That Work and Those That Don't, Family Planning Resources Center, 1971 ($.25).

This pamphlet gives clear, concise descriptions of common methods of birth control with information about their reliability. Helpfully illustrated. Available by mail from 44 Court Street, Brooklyn, New York 11201.

Love, Sex and Being Human, Paul Hobannan. Doubleday, 1969 (paper, $1.45).

This brief volume contains an excellent presentation of the physiological and emotional aspects of sexual growth and the moral and ethical dilemmas that face the sexually mature person.

Sex is For Real: Human Sexuality and Sexual Responsibility, Willard Dalrymple. McGraw-Hill, 1969 ($5.95).

This book encompasses every aspect of human sexuality, from anatomical biology to sociological, psychological, and philosophical issues involved in responsible decision making. Since it includes discussions of marriage and sex education for children, it is also profitable reading for parents. Illustrated.

Conception, Birth, and Contraception, Robert Demarest and John Sciarra. McGraw-Hill, 1969 ($8.95).

Although there is no attempt here to deal with the emotional aspects of sex and reproduction, this book is an excellent pictorial, scientific presentation of the subject.

Honest Sex, Della Roy and Rustúm Roy. New American Library, 1969 (pap., $.95).

Index to Questions

Introduction: Sex Education in A Changing World

What are my own feelings about sex?   7
What do I feel about myself?   8
What do I think about sex?   8

I. The Early Years

When does sex begin?   13
What does baby learn first?   13
Can an unhappy experience at this age do permanent damage?   14
Should baby be stopped from putting everything in his mouth?   14
When does sucking stop?   15
Is masturbation dangerous?   16
What about toilet training?   17
When is he ready to start?   18
Must we use "scientific" words?   18
Should a child see his parents nude?   18
Should I let my child into the bathroom with me?   19
Does it help to use examples of sex in nature?   19
Does the father have a place in sex education?   20
What if there is no father in the home?   20
How can I talk about sex comfortably?   21
What are some of the questions preschool children ask?   22
    How does the baby breathe inside the mother?   24
    How does the baby go to the bathroom inside the mother? 24
    Where does the baby come out?   24

Does it hurt to have a baby?   25
Why can't men have babies?   25
Why do women have breasts?   25
What if a child never asks questions about sex?   25

II. *Your Child from Five to Eight*

What are some of the questions children five to eight ask?   30
  How does a baby get inside the mother?   30
  Is semen the same as urine?   31
  Why does the mother get so big?   31
  How big is the baby when he's born?   31
Should fathers as well as mothers be involved in sex education?   32
Should children share a bed or a bedroom?   32
Should children be told about molesters?   33
What is the parent's role during the five-to-eight period?   33

IV. *Preadolescence: Ages Nine to Twelve*

What about masturbation?   47
What should preadolescents know about sexual development?   47
What is menstruation?   48
Does ovulation or menstruation hurt?   49
Why do boys have wet dreams?   50
How do the male organs of sex and reproduction work?   50
How does the cell turn into a baby?   51
Does a baby start every time people mate?   51
Why does a baby look like its parents?   51
What causes twins?   52
What causes birth defects?   52

V. *The Adolescent Years: Ages Thirteen to Seventeen*

How do physical changes affect the developing identity of young
  people?   57

How do parents deal with young people whose clothes or hair-styles seem too bizarre? 58

Why are peers so important to adolescents? 60

How do adolescents find their own way? 61

Should teenagers go steady? 62

Should petting be discouraged? 63

Does information about contraception encourage adolescents to engage in sexual intercourse? 65

What are the currently available contraceptive methods? 66

Why do girls continue to become pregnant when contraceptives are effective and available? 69

What about abortion? 71

What about venereal diseases? 73

What are the symptoms? 74

What is homosexuality? 76

What attitude can a parent reasonably assume about premarital intercourse? 79